Getting into

Dental School

Adam Cross and Emily Lucas

12th edition

trotman | t

Getting into guides

Getting into Art & Design Courses, 11th edition
Getting into Business & Economics Courses, 14th edition
Getting into Dental School, 12th edition
Getting into Engineering Courses, 6th edition
Getting into Law, 13th edition
Getting into Medical School: 2022 Entry, 26th edition
Getting into Oxford & Cambridge: 2022 Entry, 24th edition
Getting into Pharmacy and Pharmacology Courses, 2nd edition
Getting into Physiotherapy Courses, 10th edition
Getting into Psychology Courses, 13th edition
Getting into Veterinary School, 12th edition
How to Complete Your UCAS Application: 2022 Entry, 33rd edition

Getting into Dental School

This 12th edition published in 2021 by Trotman Education, an imprint of Trotman Publishing Ltd, 21d Charles Street, Bath BA1 1HX

© Trotman Publishing Ltd 2021

Authors: Adam Cross and Emily Lucas

7th–11th edns: Adam Cross
6th edn: Steven Piumatti
5th edn: James Burnett
3rd & 4th edns: James Burnett & Andrew Long
2nd edn: Joe Ruston & James Burnett
1st edn: Joe Ruston
Editions 1–4 published by Trotman and Co. Ltd

British Library Cataloguing in Publication Data
A catalogue record of this book is available from the British Library.

ISBN: 978 1 912943 34 0

Printed and bound in the UK by Ashford Colour Press Ltd

Contents

About the authors   v

Acknowledgements   vi

Introduction   1
What role do dentists have in society?   2
What are the necessary attributes of a dentist?   5
Are there any downsides to being a dentist?   6

1| **Studying dentistry**   **8**
Exploring the options   10
University courses   13
Undergraduate   14
Postgraduate   21

2| **Getting work experience**   **24**
How to arrange work experience   25
Things to look out for during work experience   26
The importance of voluntary work   29
Making the most of your work experience and voluntary work   29
Work experience and voluntary work during the pandemic   32

3| **Choosing your course**   **34**
Choice of school   34
Open days   36
Non-academic considerations   37
Academic requirements   37
The impact of Covid-19 on dental school places   42
The UCAS Tariff   43
Other qualifications   43
Non-dental choices   44

4| **The UCAS application**   **47**
UCAS Apply   47
When to submit your UCAS application   48
The reference   48
UCAT   49
BMAT   66
Deferred entry   72
Dental timeline   72

5| **Personal statement**   **74**
Personal statement basics   75
Sections of the personal statement   75

Weak and strong personal statements 79
Application checklist 87
What happens next? 88

6| What makes a successful interview? **89**
Multiple mini interviews 89
Panel interviews 94
Questions to reflect on in preparation for your interview 94
How to succeed in the interview 102
At the end of your interview 102
General interview tips 103
How you are selected 104
What happens next? 105
Current issues in dentistry 105

7| Non-standard applications **121**
Those who have not studied science at A level 121
Overseas students 122
Mature students 125
Studying abroad 130
Students with disabilities and special educational needs 134

8| What do I do on results day? **135**
If things go wrong during the exams 135
If you hold an offer and get the grades 136
If you hold no offer 136
If you hold an offer but miss the grades 138
Retaking A levels 139
Reapplying to dental school 142

9| Fees and funding **145**
Fees 146
Financial help 148

10| What career pathways exist for dentists? **152**
General dental practitioners (GDPs) 152
Hospital and community dentists 155
Dental specialisms 155
Other careers in dentistry 158
Running a business 159
The wider team 159
Salaries and wages 160
Graduate prospects 162

11| Further information **165**
Further reading 165
Organisations 166
Dental schools 166

Glossary **169**

About the authors

Adam Cross is Vice Principal at the independent college MPW Birmingham and has a number of years' expertise in helping students gain entry onto highly competitive undergraduate courses such as dentistry and medicine. In addition to his UCAS and careers guidance expertise, Adam also helps students with pre-admissions tests such as the University Clinical Aptitude Test (UCAT) and BioMedical Admissions Test (BMAT). Adam studied Biological Sciences at Lancaster University and currently teaches A level Biology at MPW. He is also co-author of Trotman's *Getting into Medical School* guide.

Emily Lucas read Medical Science at the University of Birmingham before obtaining a master's degree in Genomic Medicine at Queen Mary, University of London. She currently holds the position of University Support Officer and helps students with their university applications, as well as supporting students with pre-admissions tests such as the University Clinical Aptitude Test (UCAT) and the BioMedical Admissions Test (BMAT). As well as teaching, Emily has maintained a research position at the University of Birmingham in the field of epigenetics. Emily also teaches biology, and is the current author of Trotman's *Getting into Law* and *Getting into Veterinary School* guides, as well as being co-author of *Getting into Medical School*.

Acknowledgements

We would like to thank all of the individuals who have given their time to provide information about their experiences of studying dentistry and working as a dentist. In particular, we would like to thank Yusra Khan, Simran Chahal, Maisie Shay, Shyam Patel, Andy Shaw, Hamza Khan, Sumandeep Kailey and Avani Gill for taking the time to reflect on their experiences of studying dentistry and providing us with an insight into the life of a dental student. We would like to thank Dr Ayesha Mohammed, Dr Suraj Bath, Dr Khaleda Shah and Dr Sameera Mukadam for providing an insight into the working world of a dentist. We would also like to thank Hamza Khan and Andy Shaw for allowing us to reproduce their personal statements in the book, which led to successful entry onto dentistry programmes this year.

In addition, we would like to thank the admissions teams from all of the UK dental schools, the British Dental Association and the British Dental Health Foundation for providing material relating to the world of dentistry.

Introduction

If you have picked up this book, you are probably considering applying to study dentistry and ultimately want to become a dentist. At this stage of the process, you may be unsure about the details of how to apply, or how best to prepare yourself for an admissions interview. You may have no idea about the type of work experience you will be required to have or the demands of pre-admissions tests. However, the whole purpose of this book is to provide you with a step-by-step guide to the whole process and ensure that you are prepared to make a successful application and secure your place at university.

This book is divided into the following chapters, which will guide you through each stage of the process.

Chapter 1 gives an overview of studying dentistry at university and describes the experiences you will have as an undergraduate and the key elements of the course structure. It then explores options for post-graduate study and the various specialisms that exist.

Chapter 2 outlines the importance of work experience and voluntary work when making your application and the areas for you to focus on to maximise your chances of successfully applying.

Chapter 3 includes advice on what to consider when choosing the course you wish to apply to. It looks in particular at what to consider when attending open days and the various academic requirements that the courses have.

Chapter 4 deals with preparing your application to make it as attractive as possible to admissions tutors. It includes advice on the UCAS application procedure and also deals with the University Clinical Aptitude Test (UCAT) and BioMedical Admissions Test (BMAT) and how best to prepare for them.

Chapter 5 focuses on the personal statement and how to write it. It looks at the general structure of the statement and the elements that need to be included to make you stand out.

Chapter 6 provides advice on how to prepare for multiple mini interviews (MMIs) and panel interviews. It also gives some examples of the types of questions that you may be asked. It goes on to provide key information on some current dental issues, such as mouth cancer, fluoridation of water and NHS dentistry.

Chapter 7 gives information about international students applying to study dentistry, but also deals with applications from other non-standard applicants, such as mature students, graduates, students who have studied arts A levels, and retake students.

Chapter 8 looks at the options you have on results day and describes the steps that you need to take if you miss the grades or do not hold any offers.

Chapter 9 looks at the financial elements of being a dental student and gives details of fees, student loans and grants across the UK.

Chapter 10 looks at career options in dentistry and the different pathways that a dentist could follow. It also looks at your graduate prospects as a dentist and what typical earnings are.

Finally, in **Chapter 11**, you can find details of all the dental schools and key dental organisations, plus a glossary that can be used to decipher any technical terms you come across.

There are a number of case studies provided throughout the book to support the material being discussed. This information is designed to illustrate the appropriate points and should give you an opportunity to see the issues under consideration demonstrated. Like other books in this series, such as *Getting into Medical School*, this title is designed to be a route map for potential dentists rather than a guide to dentistry as a profession. Further information on issues relating to being a dentist can be found on websites such as the British Dental Association's (the BDA – see www.bda.org), or directly from your own dentist.

Entrance requirements have been given primarily in terms of A level grades throughout the book; information for students who have studied Scottish Highers, the International Baccalaureate (IB) and other qualifications is given in Chapter 3.

What role do dentists have in society?

When researching the profession, most prospective dentists soon realise that it involves much more than gazing into people's mouths all day! It is a challenging vocation that requires a wide range of scientific and personal skills to be mastered in order to be successful.

So why do so many people aspire to study dentistry? Dental professionals often cite a number of positive aspects to pursuing dentistry as a career, which include:

- developing your interest in human anatomy, particularly in relation to the head and mouth
- helping to improve the oral health and confidence of a wide range of people from a range of backgrounds
- being a positive and active member of the local community
- working with your hands, and being able to demonstrate high levels of manual dexterity

- interacting with a wide range of people on a day-to-day basis
- running a business and being your own boss
- flexibility in working hours
- working as part of a team.

Some dentists may also cite the financial benefits and the status and respect that go hand in hand with the career. However, while these factors may play some part in your decision to pursue a career in dentistry, they are certainly not good enough reasons on their own, and would undoubtedly have a negative impact on your application were they ever conveyed to an admissions team.

One of the major focuses of modern dentistry is about general oral health. Dentists are increasingly occupying a much wider societal role than they once had; in addition to carrying out standard treatments, as oral professionals and health practitioners they look after the well-being of their patients and thus become an important part of any community. For example, a dentist may give advice on diet, giving up smoking and its possible knock-on effects for general health, as well as recommendations about courses of dental treatment.

The Oral Health Foundation has an interesting website, www.dental health.org, which outlines the variety of issues that dentists must consider when treating patients on a daily basis. These include obvious concerns such as dental decay and sensitive teeth, but also more wide-ranging themes such as mouth cancer, diet and bad breath. A quick look through this site should give you an insight into a number of these problems.

In addition to a comprehensive knowledge of the scientific and technical foundation of dentistry, dentists must also have the interpersonal skills required to deal with a wide variety of patients, including those with additional needs. This can pose unique challenges for a dentist; those with physical disabilities may need assistance to get into the dental chair, while people with learning disabilities may become distressed at the thought of going to the dentist and require extra time to be reassured and appropriately cared for. Some patients may have other special needs, such as communication difficulties or being visually or hearing impaired. People with severe medical problems may also need extra care in order to be treated safely and successfully. A dentist must take account of all these and have the skills to deal with them when providing dental care. A dentist may even have to make different arrangements to meet the needs of the individual, and often home visits will need to be organised. Community dental services in the UK currently provide treatment of both old and young people with special medical or social needs, such as complex medical problems, disabilities or mental health problems, who cannot be treated by general dental practitioners (GDPs).

Another major aspect of the role that dentists have in society is education. Along with dental nurses they are at the forefront of teaching the public about good dental hygiene. One of the primary focuses in modern dentistry is on preventive dentistry which aims to promote long-term care of the mouth, teeth, gums and cheeks, and extends, as mentioned earlier, to advice on areas such as diet and lifestyle. Teaching awareness of oral health and hygiene is of paramount importance. Dentists educate patients on caring for their teeth and gums by encouraging them to use a brush with the correct technique, to floss and to use the correct products. Teaching through direct consultations or via literature available in surgeries are just some of the ways that this can be achieved; other ways include the education of young people in schools, and educating elderly people in nursing homes about keeping dentures clean and viable.

Ultimately, the goal of educating the population about oral health and preventive dentistry is to keep the need for major dental treatment to a minimum by maintaining a healthy mouth. The two major causes of tooth loss are tooth decay and gum disease, so the successful prevention of these two problems massively increases the probability of an individual keeping their teeth for life. The joint efforts of the dentist, the hygienist and the patient can help to prevent the need for treatment, and so avoid the pattern of fillings and extractions. This is a saving not only to the individual in terms of time and money but also to the community in the long term.

Dentists can often be the first to spot medical issues that might otherwise go unnoticed until the problem has worsened. One example of this is oral cancer. The most recent published statistics show that there are approximately 12,200 new cases of head and neck cancer each year (this figure accounts for all forms of oral cancer between 2015 and 2017), with approximately 4,000 patients dying from the disease (www.cancerresearchuk.org/health-professional/cancer-statistics/statistics-by-cancer-type/head-and-neck-cancers/incidence#heading-Zero). The role of the dentist is therefore vital in early diagnosis and referral for appropriate treatment. Dentists are also the first people to recognise other problems, such as ulcers and cold sores, which could lead to more serious conditions. As with all disease, early recognition is more than half the battle.

Cosmetic dentistry is a huge industry, with dentists playing a role in providing treatments to straighten, lighten, reshape and repair teeth. Such treatments can include providing veneers, crowns, bridges, tooth-coloured fillings, implants, tooth whitening and correction of bites. Usually abnormal 'bites' or crooked teeth are fixed in childhood, but today even mild abnormalities that have been previously left untreated are seen as a problem and as a consequence more young and mature adults than before are undergoing this type of treatment. The demand for cosmetic treatments continues to grow, due in part to the desire for a flawless smile and, as a result, is a lucrative area for dentists to become involved in.

What are the necessary attributes of a dentist?

As with any highly competitive university course and vocation, in order to succeed candidates must be able to demonstrate their academic ability, the right personal qualities, plus commitment. Practising dentists, admissions tutors and current students all agree that showing genuine dedication to dentistry is essential during the application process, university study and beyond into a dentist's professional life.

It is therefore vital that an applicant to dentistry is certain that they want to be a dentist before applying. Wanting to study dentistry because 'you like science' or because 'you want a job with high employment rates' will not convince an admissions tutor to give you a place. It is also unlikely to be enough to keep you motivated throughout your working life.

Dentistry, unlike medicine, offers fewer diverse pathways or opportunities later on in your career. This ultimately means that you must be fully informed about what the career path entails because it is difficult to move into something else without some degree of re-specialisation.

In addition to being fully committed to dentistry, a dentist must also be able to demonstrate the following:

- the ability to successfully communicate with patients
- an enjoyment in dealing with people and working in a team
- an ability to reassure patients who are scared or in pain
- a caring and sympathetic nature and immense patience
- a high degree of manual dexterity
- self-motivation
- an enjoyment of science
- an interest in current issues in relation to dentistry and oral health
- an excellent memory and an ability to solve problems
- versatility
- mental and physical stamina
- the ability to multi-task between clinical work and the business side of running a practice
- an ability to train and manage people and get the best out of them.

Most of the above qualities should not surprise you. It would be hard to be a successful dentist if you could not bear to be around other people, and unsympathetic dentists end up with few patients. Similarly, if you do not enjoy science, you would be unlikely to gain the necessary grades at A level or pass your exams at university. But often overlooked is the need for stamina when carrying out long and repetitive procedures; concentrating on one thing for hours might not be for you if you struggle to maintain concentration!

If you believe that you have at least some of the qualities listed above, the next step is to investigate what being a dentist is actually like and to find out what a dentist does. In brief, a dentist's job can include a range of tasks, for example carrying out routine examinations, filling cavities, examining X-rays, applying protective sealant on teeth, extracting teeth, removing decay, fitting dental implants, taking measurements and making models for dentures. This gives a small glimpse into the versatility needed by a practising dentist.

Many people are unaware that dentists are usually self-employed, and the amount of money they earn is directly related to the number of patients they see. Without stamina and self-motivation, as well as some degree of business acumen, you are unlikely to earn as much as you might hope.

Research released in October 2020 estimated the average debt of students finishing their courses in 2019 at £40,000 (https://commons library.parliament.uk/research-briefings/sn01079). While studying at university, many students accrue multiple debts, including student loans (tuition fee and maintenance loans), overdrafts, credit cards, debts to parents and sometimes even commercial loans. Therefore, once qualified, dentists need to earn enough not only to support themselves but also to begin paying off these debts. It should also be remembered that the average student debt figure of £40,000 is largely based on three-year degree courses, so the average figure for a dental student is likely to be even higher.

As part of the government's Teaching Excellence Framework (TEF), which ranks English universities and colleges based on the quality of their teaching, universities that have a TEF award can charge up to the maximum amount (£9,250). Universities without a TEF award can only charge up to £9,000 per year. It is likely that student fees will continue to rise in line with inflation in coming years, so levels of student debt are expected to continue to rise.

Are there any downsides to being a dentist?

There are, of course, some negative aspects of dentistry. Some of the common downsides that dentists cite relate to issues including stress, the demanding nature of being self-employed, lack of career progression, aggressive or frightened patients, and, last but by no means least, the boredom that can accompany repetitive routine tasks. If you are worried about any of these, you should talk to your own dentist to see how he or she feels about them.

Before looking at the applications and admissions processes in more detail, you may be interested to read what a current dental student had to say about her choice of career thus far. Bear in mind that this could be you in one or two years' time.

Case study: Yusra Khan, first-year dentistry student

'My interest in pursuing a career in dentistry began while visiting family abroad. I observed the lack of dental hygiene and an absence in preventative measures especially in school-aged children, which contrasted with dentistry in the UK. I noticed that there were many disparities within local areas, and often dental care was not up to par. This led me to want to educate parents and children in my area. I started distributing information leaflets about brushing techniques and how to prevent caries. When I returned home, I decided that I wanted to carry on pursuing the same goals of improving oral health in the UK.

'Prior to applying, I undertook work experience for three weeks in a dental practice and for one week in an orthodontic and maxillo-facial clinic at a hospital. I was also able to witness an extraction under general anaesthetic. From this work experience, I learnt a variety of transferable skills from both the dentist and the dental nurse. I was particularly impressed by the techniques used when managing an anxious patient and the steps that must be put in place when a patient has additional needs.

'My journey to securing my place to study dentistry was a tough one, but through perseverance and dedication I was able to secure the grades I needed to study at the University of Leeds. Since starting the course, I have particularly enjoyed learning something new each day and that I have been able to build step-by-step on the foundation I laid during A levels.

'My tips for prospective students are:
- be prepared for long days at university and a heavy workload
- much of the work in some modules is self-taught, so be ready to go out and research tasks independently – you won't get everything spoon-fed to you
- find a great group of friends who have a similar mindset to you and enjoy your time in university!'

1 | Studying dentistry

According to UCAS, in 2019 there were 11,450 applicants for entry onto dentistry courses competing for 1,140 places, a ratio of 10 applications per place. In terms of gender, there were approximately 16 women securing a place for every 9 men. Male applicants had a slightly lower success rate of 9%, compared to 10% for female applicants. It is clear from scrutinising the application statistics over the last eight years that there are some significant patterns in dentistry applications related to gender; there have consistently been more applications and more places gained by females in comparison with their male counterparts (see Table 1 opposite). There are undoubtedly numerous reasons behind this, but it seems this is a sustained pattern that is not just due to chance.

Around 420 of the total number of applicants were from the EU (excluding the UK), with only 10 being accepted, which represents a success rate of just 2%. For other non-EU international students, there were 875 applicants, with only 85 being accepted, a success rate of just under 10%. This demonstrates that it is far more difficult for your application to be successful if you are an overseas applicant, and the reasons for this are discussed further in Chapter 7.

In recent years, it has become obvious that total applicant numbers for dentistry have been steadily declining; since 2010, there has been a 14% decrease in applications (see Table 1). However, there was an increase of 16% in overall applications between 2018 and 2019. One of the most noticeable statistics in relation to the fall in applicants is that it has been largely driven by fewer men applying; since 2010, male applications have fallen 24%, while female applications have decreased by 3%.

There are likely to be a number of factors that have caused this dip in numbers, with the most important one likely being the introduction of £9,000 tuition fees in 2012. However, despite this decrease in numbers, it is clear that there is still an extremely strong demand for places on dental courses and the success rates are still relatively low. Prospective dental students should therefore ensure that they are not lulled into a false sense of security; a dip in applications does not mean significantly easier entry! As has always been the case, top grades and thorough preparation are irreplaceable when trying to make a successful application.

Table 1 UCAS End of Cycle Applicant statistics for dentistry – 2010–19 (most recent published data)

Year	Applications	Places	Applications per place	Male applications	Males gaining places	Female applications	Females gaining places	Male success rate	Female success rate	Overseas applications (EU/Non-EU)
2019	11450	1140	9.96	4390	415	7060	725	9%	10%	420/875
2018	9850	1125	8.76	3800	420	6050	705	11%	12%	335/960
2017	9240	1135	8.14	3565	415	5675	720	12%	13%	365/1050
2016	9060	1100	8.24	3575	430	5485	670	12%	12%	465/1160
2015	9875	1095	9.02	3920	410	5960	685	10%	11%	490/1320
2014	11210	1100	10.14	4360	395	6850	705	9%	10%	515/1225
2013	11350	1185	9.54	4725	460	6625	725	10%	11%	635/1100
2012	11630	1195	9.73	5010	470	6615	725	9%	11%	600/1185
2011	12550	1195	10.50	5670	510	6880	685	9%	10%	775/1170
2010	13055	1280	10.20	5790	525	7268	755	9%	10%	905/1020
% change 2018–19	+16%	+1%	+14%	+16%	−1%	+17%	+3%			
% change 2010–19	−14%	−12%	−2%	−24%	−21%	−3%	−4%			

Source: www.ucas.com/data-and-analysis/ucas-undergraduate-releases/ucas-undergraduate-end-cycle-data-resources.
We acknowledge UCAS' contribution of this information.

Exploring the options

So what are the steps that you need to take to ensure that you have an excellent chance of being selected for an interview and offered a place?

The first step is to thoroughly research the stages of the application process and the demands of the course and career. This is vital for a number of reasons. You need to:

- see whether dentistry is the right career for you
- see whether your personal and academic skills are matched to the course
- find out which universities offer dentistry and to which you want to apply
- find out the details of courses offered by each university and the one that might best suit you (while the courses may have the same title, their structures can differ)
- find out the academic requirements for the course and which pre-admissions test is needed
- gain ideas and information about possible work experience placements
- find out what makes an excellent personal statement
- understand the demands of the interview process and develop interview skills.

Ideally, your research should start in the first year of your A levels (Fifth year in Scotland) or even earlier; the most committed prospective dentists I meet often start their preparation in year 10 or before. Most schools start a programme of UCAS and career prospects-related workshops halfway through the first year of A levels, with the aim being that students should have a clear idea about where they want to apply after the summer holidays. However, you should make your mind up about studying dentistry as soon as possible to give you the maximum amount of time for research and work experience placements.

There are several sources that can be used for research. These can be divided into:

- media research: internet, books, prospectuses and specialist magazines
- discussion with professionals
- work experience.

Some suggestions for media research are given below.

Internet

There are a wide variety of resources available on the internet that are useful for researching the profession and for preparing for interviews.

- The UCAS website (www.ucas.com) is initially the most useful for research into degree courses and gives comprehensive details about the entry requirements and course structure at each university.
- Newspaper sites: the *Guardian* (www.theguardian.com/education/universityguide) and the *Times* (www.thetimes.co.uk) provide useful information about university league tables and subject rankings. NB The *Times* can only be accessed via a subscription.
- The British Dental Association (www.bda.org) gives information primarily on topical issues for healthcare professionals.
- The Oral Health Foundation (www.dentalhealth.org) focuses more on raising public awareness of important oral hygiene issues. This website is useful if you want to gain a wider understanding of public health issues in relation to dentistry.
- www.dentistry.co.uk and www.the-dentist.co.uk are very useful online periodicals offering up-to-date information.
- News websites: sites like the BBC news website (www.bbc.co.uk/news) have up-to-date articles about current affairs related to dentistry and health.
- University websites: most of the information you will need about applying to a university and about the course can be found on individual universities' websites. These are a treasure trove of information and will help you get a feel for each institution and the nature of the course it is offering.
- The Complete University Guide (www.thecompleteuniversityguide.co.uk) and Discover Uni (https://discoveruni.gov.uk) websites provide impartial information relating to universities and courses. These are useful resources to help find out information relating to student feedback, satisfaction scores and employment rates.

Books, magazines and prospectuses

- *HEAP 2021: University Degree Course Offers* by Brian Heap has a short section on dentistry and the universities offering dentistry courses, and gives a good overview of entry requirements.
- University prospectuses: visiting each university website and requesting a prospectus will help you get a feel for the institution and the course. Note that a number of universities have full prospectuses online.
- Subscribing to magazines such as *The Dentist* will let you find out first-hand about issues and developments in dentistry. This would be seen as extracurricular reading and would demonstrate your interest to university admissions panels.

Case study: Simran Chahal

'I chose to study dentistry because it was a career that I was really passionate about following my work experience. During my GCSEs, I was totally adamant that I wanted to be a lawyer and hence chose to do my work experience placement in a law firm. It was a life lesson for sure! I didn't enjoy it one bit and went back to the drawing board, I looked at what I enjoyed at school and where my strengths were. I looked into dentistry following the recommendations of some of my friends that had already applied to university and decided to carry out some work experience within the field.

'It wasn't just the skills required for the profession that drew me in but the fact that you are able to meet so many people each day, each with their own stories and backgrounds. Furthermore, dentistry is a career that doesn't ever end, throughout your life you will always be learning as the industry develops, and this is something that really excites me! My job will never get boring! When you begin to study dentistry you will soon come to realise that there are numerous area of specialisation and options for branching out into different fields.

'Working in clinics in deprived areas of the country has brought to light the impact that "simple" procedures, such as scaling and polishing, can have on patients, and how improved oral health can potentially change an individual's life.

'Before applying, I carried out a bulk of my work experience during my first year of A levels over a prolonged period at a local practice. Additionally, I was able to shadow in the oral maxillofacial department at a hospital in Birmingham.

'My placement in the dental surgery showed me how important teamwork is; if there isn't a nurse present a lot of disruption is caused. It has become even more apparent since starting my own training. I also saw how empathy and being non-judgemental were of vital importance; there could be a number of factors that contribute to the state of a person's oral hygiene and so it is important not to jump to conclusions.

'Since starting my course, I have had to work really hard, but have also had lots of rewarding experiences. A lot of people on my course found the jump between A levels and undergraduate study tough. You have to become independent, motivate yourself to do the best and stay on top of your study. At the end of my first year I treated several patients and carried out a large number of clinical procedures on the phantom heads. These next few years excite me as I will slowly become more capable of carrying out clinical procedures and be able to treat an increasing number of people!

'The clinical aspect of the course is by far the most enjoyable and makes the 8 a.m. starts worthwhile. As a student you are able to spend a lot longer with patients, meaning that you are able to get to know them as a person and build a relationship with them. The hardest part is when it comes to summer or a referral and you have to discharge them!

'In terms of challenges, I find it difficult to make time for my friends outside of the course, because they have a lot more free time and you can't always afford to socialise with them until late in the evening or you're just too tired to even go out! However, it does get easier as you adjust to a new routine and find a balance.

'My tips for aspiring dentists are:
- ensure you stay on top of study from the start, it will help you so much when it comes to exams
- try and improve your manual dexterity skills before you start university
- if you're looking to apply to university, have a look at when they start clinics and actually treat patients; some universities start later than others and you could wait three years to realise that you don't like the job at all
- don't be put off by the interview process
- be prepared for long hours
- get plenty of experience in as many aspects as you can.'

University courses

In the UK, the General Dental Council (GDC) publishes a document that outlines the requirements of all dental programmes leading to GDC registration. These 'Standards for Education' (www.gdc-uk.org/education-cpd/quality-assurance) ensure that all dental schools have to deal with a prescribed set of learning outcomes over the duration of the course. This means that there is a significant degree of similarity between the dental courses offered at different universities. However, it is also vital to remember that different dental schools will have different ways of approaching these outcomes, and consequently course structure and teaching approaches may differ greatly; this can ultimately result in massively different experiences for students when studying dentistry. It is therefore vital that you thoroughly research how each course is structured so that they can truly understand what it will be like to study dentistry at a particular university. This section therefore aims to give you some idea of the key things you will experience as a dental student throughout the duration of your studies.

Undergraduate

Studying dentistry in the UK is a challenging but highly rewarding experience, and the provision at British dental schools is normally first rate. Prospective students should be aware from the outset that undertaking this course will require commitment and dedication; ask any current dental student and they will tell you how much hard work is needed to succeed. Undergraduate dental courses last for five years and at the end of their studies students will gain the initials BDS or BChD (the Latin equivalent of BDS) after their name. There is no distinction between these two classifications as both refer to a Bachelor of Dental Surgery; the distinction depends on the dental school that a student has attended.

As outlined above, most of the dental schools have a similar structure in their courses but key differences have begun to emerge in the teaching methodology and delivery of course content. It is therefore important for students to carefully research the details of each course and appreciate the key features. This is obviously vital in selecting an appropriate dental school, submitting a relevant personal statement and preparing for an interview. Many of the dental schools have started to put a greater emphasis on students taking responsibility for their own learning. At Leeds, for example, much emphasis is placed on clinical dentistry throughout the course, with first clinical exposure occurring in year 1.

Integrated learning, problem-based learning (PBL) and enquiry-based learning (EBL)

Universities teach in a range of ways, from traditional large lectures to small tuition groups; however, most faculties employ a wide range of methods to ensure their students develop into highly competent practitioners. Some schools, such as Liverpool, have successfully developed courses that have some elements of problem-based learning (PBL) at their core. Many of the dental schools have begun to place a greater responsibility on students to be accountable for their own learning, and prospective students should be aware of terms such as enquiry-based learning (EBL), self-directed learning and computer-based learning.

These approaches are designed to develop an independent and inquisitive approach to learning, using libraries and discussing issues with colleagues to solve problems (as the name suggests). Bristol, by contrast, does not explicitly use the PBL approach, and adopts a system based on lectures, workshops, tutorials and practical sessions. Many courses integrate elements of clinical contact from the first year of the course, while others do not introduce clinical contact until year two. At Birmingham and Cardiff, for example, first-year students will have exposure to clinical contact, whereas at Bristol and Plymouth, clinical teaching and patient treatment begin in the second year. As you would expect, all dental schools are committed to using up-to-date technology to help teach the curriculum, and students will notice how keen the various dental schools are to demonstrate this during open days.

Course structure

Year one

The reason why a dental course lasts five years is that the teaching covers a wide variety of elements. All dental schools will offer one or two years of pre-clinical study that lays the biological foundation for the rest of the course and clinical practice. This is often taught outside the school and covers numerous themes such as:

- anatomy
- oral health and disease
- biochemistry
- physiology
- biochemistry
- microbiology
- oral biology
- cell biology.

In addition, students will often cover introductory modules related to communication, interpersonal skills, clinical competence and teamworking skills, due to the patient-centred nature of the profession. Many dental schools will also introduce some limited clinical exposure in the first year.

Years two to five

As the course progresses, the amount of clinical work that you carry out will increase, with most universities offering increased levels of clinical contact from the second year. Alongside your clinical and skill development work, you will continue with programmes in areas such as oral biology, disease and pathology. You will also learn about the social and psychological aspects of patient care while developing your interpersonal and communication skills.

As the clinical part of the course increases in importance, students will usually take responsibility for their own patients. During the third year of the programme at Birmingham, for example, students are given responsibility for their own patients' treatment in what amounts to their own mini-practice in the dental hospital. Students will also spend time in other settings, such as dental access centres, general dental practices or community practices to gain practical experience. Some courses involve spending time in local hospitals to gain experience of the secondary care that takes place following a referral from a dentist. In order to teach the patient care necessary to treat a range of people effectively, there may be modules in behavioural sciences and the management of pain and anxiety, as well as in the treatment of children, the elderly and disabled people. Clinical students will typically study some of the following courses (full details of each course can be found on individual university websites):

- dental materials science
- dental public health
- haematology
- operative technique and clinical skills
- paediatric dentistry
- restorative dentistry
- oral medicine and surgery
- oral pathology
- oral biochemistry and biology
- oral diseases
- orthodontics
- endodontics
- prosthodontics
- periodontics
- pharmacology
- nutrition and diet
- medico-legal and ethical aspects of dental practice
- forensic dentistry
- sedation
- behavioural science
- oral radiography
- communication skills
- management and leadership
- social and behavioural science.

Some universities offer their students the opportunity to complete an intercalated BSc. This is normally a one-year project, during which time you pause your dentistry degree and investigate a chosen topic in much more depth. This usually results in securing an additional degree before rejoining the course the following year.

Your final years of study consist primarily of further development of clinical skills to consolidate the knowledge and skills that you have previously acquired and prepare you for practising once you have qualified. You will continue to have extensive and varied clinical exposure in a number of settings outside of the dental school throughout this time. There is also further academic work that continues alongside the practical components. As you near the end of your clinical course, you may have time to pursue your own elective programme of study – a topic of personal interest, which you research on your own.

At the end of year five, there is the final BDS/BChD professional examination. On successful completion of the course, graduates are competent to carry out most treatments and exercise independent clinical judgement.

Two examples of course outlines are provided in the boxes below to illustrate the common threads and differences between different universities.

Programme structure: University of Plymouth (2019)

You will treat patients through partnership with Peninsula Dental Social Enterprise and the wider NHS in Devon and Cornwall, become familiar with a variety of clinical situations, and prepare for a future career path through solving clinical problems. You'll also discover how clinical dentistry and research is practised in different social and cultural contexts in other parts of the South-west, the rest of the UK and across the world.

Year 1

Your clinical education commences at the start of Year 1, working in small, integrated study groups you will learn the core scientific foundations of dentistry in a clinical context, explore the scientific basis of normal structure, function and behaviour, with a focus on dental health, prevention of dental disease and the underlying principles of personal and professional development. You will attend the Simulated Dental Learning Environment (SDLE) from your first week, developing essential clinical skills. In Term 2 you will experience contact with patients in the clinics, where you will be able to develop your communication skills under the close supervision of dental practitioners, bringing to life the skills gained in SDLE. Near the end of the year you have your first experience in social engagement.

Core modules

- DEN411 Integrated Dental Science 1
- DEN412 Clinical Dental Practice 1
- DEN413 Clinical Dental Practice 2
- DEN414 Inter-Professional Engagement 1
- DEN415 Professional Development 1

Year 2

In your second year, you build on your foundations with common dental problems, as well as disease mechanisms considered in much greater depth. Learning continues in SDLE as you develop skills for advanced procedures while continuing to care for patients

---

in the clinics in Plymouth two days per week. You gain insight into the importance of team working in dentistry as you integrate with other members of the team in the clinical environment, and plan and deliver a social engagement project intervention.

Core modules

- DEN521 Integrated Dental Science 2
- DEN522 Clinical Dental Practice 3
- DEN523 Clinical Dental Practice 4
- DEN524 Inter-Professional Engagement 2
- DEN525 Professional Development 2

Year 3

In your Year 3 there is greater self-directed learning as you prepare project assignments, including an engagement project with students from another healthcare profession, and clinical cases. Based in Plymouth, with transport provided to the Exeter clinic two days per week, you build upon existing skills and consolidate advanced procedures provided for patients. One of the themes for years three and four is to consolidate the learning of medically related issues for the safe practice of dentistry. You will be given an opportunity to learn about dentally relevant medical issues in patient-based demonstrations.

Core modules

- DEN631 Applied Dental Knowledge 1
- DEN632 Critical Appraisal 1
- DEN633 Clinical Dental Practice 5
- DEN634 Clinical Dental Practice 6
- DEN635 Inter-Professional Engagement 3
- DEN636 Professional Development 3

Intercalated Master of Science (MSc)

Selected students may intercalate, between Year 3 and Year 4, and undertake a one year MSc in the research laboratories in Plymouth.

Year 4

In your fourth year you will live in Truro for the whole academic year. Clinical activity will expand to three days per week and you start to prepare clinical cases for Finals. Clinical dentistry will now embrace all of the aspects of dental care provision expected of a qualified dentist, will give you experience in advanced restorative techniques, and strengthen your competence in treatment planning. You'll gain first-hand experience of the role and services provided by specialists in primary and secondary care, by spending time in specialist clinics such as restorative dentistry, oral surgery, oral diseases and orthodontics.

Core modules

- DEN641 Applied Dental Knowledge 2
- DEN642 Clinical Dental Practice 7
- DEN643 Inter-Professional Engagement 4
- DEN644 Professional Development 4

Final year

The emphasis in your final year is on the implementation and consolidation of the skills and abilities you have learned in previous years and is the final preparation for dental practice. You will become more confident with clinical situations, healthcare teams and the principles of professionalism; and discover advances in dentistry being developed for future practice.

Core modules

- DEN651 Applied Dental Knowledge 3
- DEN652 Clinical Dental Practice 8
- DEN653 Clinical Dental Practice 9
- DEN654 Inter-Professional Engagement 5
- DEN655 Professional Development 5

Source: www.plymouth.ac.uk/courses/undergraduate/
bds-dental-surgery.
Reprinted with kind permission of the University of Plymouth.

Programme structure: University of Manchester (2019)

The Bachelor of Dental Surgery (BDS) course will prepare you for a dentistry career through a combination of clinical study and basic and advanced dental sciences. Once you have mastered basic competencies in the skills facilities, you will move on to treating patients in both the University Dental Hospital and local outreach clinics early in the course. You will learn to work within a dental team to take a patient-centred approach to clinical care, practising in a professional, safe and ethical manner. Students are also trained to become reflective practitioners committed to lifelong learning.

Special features

Early clinical experience

You will be introduced to the clinical environment in the first semester of Year 1, enabling you to integrate theory and practice early on in the course.

Interdisciplinary learning

Learn alongside students and professionals from a range of backgrounds, including those training in complementary professions such as dental nursing and therapy.

Intercalation opportunities

You can study another subject to achieve a BSc award over one year between Years 2 and 3 of the BDS course.

Foundation year available

Students who do not have the required science qualifications for Year 1 entry but have achieved good grades in other non-science subjects may apply for the BDS with Foundation Year.

Course content for year 1

Basic building blocks:

- Orofacial Biology 1
- Healthy Living 1 (a healthy body)
- Team Working, Professionalism and Patient Management 1
- Patient Assessment 1

Course content for year 2

Building your knowledge, skills and attitudes:

- Orofacial Biology 2
- Healthy Living 2 (a healthy mouth)
- Team Working, Professionalism and Patient Management 2
- Patient Assessment 2
- Disease Management 2

Course content for year 3

Integrating knowledge, skills and attitudes:

- Orofacial Biology 3
- Healthy Living 3 (a healthy mind)
- Team Working, Professionalism and Patient Management 3
- Patient Assessment 3
- Disease Management 3
- Participation in the Manchester Leadership Programme (MLP)

Course content for year 4

Achieving clinical competence:

- Orofacial Biology 4
- Team Working, Professionalism and Patient Management 4
- Patient Assessment 4
- Disease Management 4

Course content for year 5

Moving to professional competence:

- Team Working, Professionalism and Patient Management 5
- Preparation for Independent Practice
- The Complex Patient

Source: www.manchester.ac.uk/study/undergraduate/courses/2021/00398/
bds-dentistry-first-year-entry/course-details/#course-profile.
Reprinted with kind permission from the University of Manchester.

Postgraduate

There are many opportunities for postgraduate study in a variety of dental subjects. It is worth noting, however, that before any form of clinical training can commence (i.e. training involving hands-on contact with patients), dental graduates must register with the GDC. Dental schools and hospitals run a wide range of postgraduate programmes that include further clinical and non-clinical training and research degree programmes. The postgraduate courses may be offered as a diploma, master's degree or doctorate and may take from one to two years, or in a few cases can be flexibly completed over a period of up to five years. Many courses are offered on a part-time basis and can therefore comfortably fit around full-time employment.

General advice and guidance is available from the Royal College of Surgeons of England (RCS) website (www.rcseng.ac.uk/dental-faculties/fds). Within this site are links to each of the universities offering postgraduate courses (www.rcseng.ac.uk/dental-faculties/fds/nacpde/postgraduate-dental-courses). If you can't find the information you need here, visit the website of the individual university directly for the most detailed, up-to-date information.

At Newcastle University, for example, there are four taught programmes. These are:

- Clinical Implant Dentistry PGDip
- Conscious Sedation PGDip
- Orthodontics MSc
- Restorative Dentistry MClinDent.

Programme details: Orthodontics at Newcastle University (2022)

The course is designed to equip you with the knowledge and skills required to complement your clinical training and aims to provide:

- knowledge to support the clinical treatment of orthodontic cases, including simple and complex cases appropriate for specialist practitioner level
- an evidence base for orthodontics and the skills required to appraise the evidence base
- applied research within orthodontics.

The course provides theoretical teaching to support the development of an orthodontic specialist. It provides a comprehensive seminar programme incorporating the theoretical and diagnostic elements of specialist knowledge, and the opportunity to carry out a research project allied to our research strategy. Our course includes:

- normal and abnormal development of the dentition
- tooth movements and facial orthopaedics
- orthodontic materials
- orthodontic biomechanics
- orthodontic techniques
- biological sciences relevant to orthodontics
- an overview of multidisciplinary orthodontics.

The aim of the research component is to expose you to the principles and practicalities of performing dental research. Projects range from laboratory studies, analysis of new data sets, systematic reviews and short-term clinical studies.

Research projects are identified and allocated during the first term. By the end of the first year you will have completed your first draft of your literature review and have established your methodology. More time is available for research during the second and third years with the dissertation handed in at the end of January of the third year. You will be encouraged to publish your research work in scientific journals.

The course, based in the School of Dental Sciences, has been running for two decades and has a good national reputation. Graduates have gone on to work in prestigious practices, senior academic posts and in hospital consultant positions.

Source: www.ncl.ac.uk/postgraduate/courses/degrees/
orthodontics-msc/#profile.
Reprinted with kind permission of Newcastle University.

Other universities are also able to provide a wide range of postgraduate options. At King's College London, for example, there are 20 taught graduate programmes, many of which can be pursued via distance learning.

While undertaking a postgraduate qualification is not mandatory, it is an excellent way to specialise in a particular area of interest. This can ultimately result in enhanced career prospects and earning potential in the long run.

In addition to the more formal postgraduate qualifications, qualified dentists are also required to participate in a specified amount of mandatory continuing professional development (CPD). This comprises short courses for qualified dentists who want to develop their knowledge of the latest methods, equipment and techniques. It is the GDC that specifies the requirements for CPD for dental professionals, and CPD is offered by numerous institutions around the country.

2| Getting work experience

Discussing your interest in dentistry with dentists working in the field is an excellent way of gathering first-hand information about the subject. It may be a good idea to start by talking to your own local dentist or any family members or friends who are dentists. Discuss with them their experiences of studying dentistry and about the career options and prospects for dentists. Remember to ask about the negative points about the profession as well as the positives, as practising dentists are the individuals who are best placed to answer these questions openly and honestly. It would also be worth asking about what they perceive to be the most relevant and interesting current issues in the world of dentistry as they are going to have the most up-to-date insight.

Following on from these initial discussions, it is then essential to organise, either by yourself or via your school, some work experience where you will be able to work-shadow a dentist and see a practice in action. Shadowing dentists is useful as it will help you to get an insight into the demands of the profession and decide whether you really want to be a dentist. You will find out what goes on in a dental surgery and some of the responsibilities that a dentist has to fulfil, as well as having an opportunity to ask questions. It will also demonstrate your commitment to admissions tutors.

It is vital to remember that undertaking relevant work placements prior to applying is now a prerequisite; it is unlikely that you will be considered unless you have evidence of two weeks' worth of experience. Even more importantly, work experience is a chance for you to decide whether dentistry is the right career for you. We have worked with numerous students who have expressed a desire to be a dentist but then totally changed their minds after a week of shadowing and observation. Conversely, we have also seen many students who have shown increased dedication to pursuing a career in dentistry following work experience.

Due to the continued competitiveness of the application process, in addition to a minimum of two weeks' work experience, it is advisable to try to demonstrate an ongoing commitment to the field of dentistry. This means that you should ideally aim to spend time with several different dentists on a regular basis over a number of months. While the basic two weeks can often be enough, anything extra will serve to strengthen your application. Preparation for your application to study dentistry must therefore start as soon as possible, preferably in the first year of your A levels (Fifth year in Scotland) or earlier; if you decide on dentistry as a career only at the start of your second A level year (Sixth year in Scotland), it will leave little or no time to build up a solid portfolio of work experience, but any insights that you are able to gain will be invaluable to your application.

How to arrange work experience

Some schools and colleges have schemes whereby they can organise work experience for you. However, where these schemes exist, it is unlikely that they will provide every placement for you, and so at some point you will have to show initiative by making the necessary arrangements. There are two routes that you should try: approaching local dentists, and making use of contacts that your friends or family may have.

In order to approach local dentists about possible work experience, you should first get the names and addresses of local dental practices from a website such as the Yellow Pages (www.yell.co.uk) or the BDA (www.bda.org). You should then write a formal email or letter, and include the name of a referee (that is, someone who can vouch for your interest in dentistry as well as your reliability). Your careers teacher, housemaster/housemistress or form teacher would be ideal as a referee. An example of a suitable email is given in the box below.

Dear Mr Littlewood [phone the practice first to find the name of the dentist you should address the email to]

I am currently in my first year of studying A levels in Biology, Chemistry, Maths and Psychology at Shuttlefield School, and I am interested in pursuing a career in dentistry. I was wondering if it would be possible to meet you to discuss what the profession is like and then perhaps spend a week shadowing you or one of your colleagues, so that I can get some first-hand experience.

If you require a reference, please contact my form tutor, Mr Jones. His contact details are as follows:

Mr T. Jones
Shuttlefield School
Shuttlefield
SH21 2CF

I look forward to hearing from you.

Yours sincerely

Robert Smith

Things to look out for during work experience

Your work experience will provide you with invaluable opportunities to develop your knowledge and understanding of dentistry as a career. It is therefore vital that you pay close attention to what is going on around you so you can get the most from the experience.

Make sure you are as professional as possible throughout your placements: dress formally and be on your best behaviour at all times. Turn your phone off and put it away so that it's not a distraction. Ask intelligent questions to further your understanding of what is going on. Offer to help the dentist or the receptionists with routine tasks. Show an interest in all that is going on around you, bearing in mind that this might be your job in a few years' time. It is also vital to buy a notebook and keep it handy during your placements. You should keep a record of:

- any procedures you observe
- any interesting, shocking or unusual cases you observe
- any reflections on your time spent shadowing.

During your placements, you should pay attention to the following aspects of dental practice.

The attributes of a dentist

Dentists need to be much more than dental treatment robots; it is therefore a good idea to keep a note of the range of characteristics the dentist demonstrates on a day-to-day basis as well as the variety of tasks they carry out. This will help provide you with a list of the sort of skills you will need to develop as a dentist and will ultimately help you in developing the knowledge of dentists you will require to write a personal statement and have a successful interview.

Interactions with patients

A vital part of the dentist's role is to interact with patients to discuss potential treatment routes and to guide and reassure them. Take time to observe how a dentist communicates with patients, particularly those who are anxious about being treated or have special needs. It is also useful to consider how a dentist might change their approach when dealing with young children compared to adults.

The variety of treatments available to patients

Make sure that you know what you are observing during your placement. Ask the dentist or nurse for the technical names of the procedures you see and for information on the materials and equipment used. Ask about the advantages and disadvantages of different types of filling, implant or denture. While you are not expected to show an in-depth understanding of every dental procedure in your application, being able to discuss a few that you have observed first-hand will demonstrate your enthusiasm and willingness to learn.

Make sure that you are aware not only of the way that damaged teeth are repaired, but also about preventive dentistry, orthodontics and oral hygiene. You should also try to discuss the dentist's role in identifying other problems, such as oral cancer.

The roles of different team members

In any dental setting, there will be a wide range of individuals involved who are vital to the overall functioning of the team. For example, in addition to the dentist there may also be dental nurses, hygienists, receptionists and administrators. Make sure you take time to talk to as many members of the team as possible and ask them about the role they play.

Working as a dentist

Ask the dentist about his or her professional life. Find out about the hours, the way in which dentists are paid, the demands of the job and the career options. Find out what dentists like about the job and what they dislike. It is important to consider the downsides to working as a dentist so that you can ascertain whether it is an appropriate career choice for you. Being able to reflect on these in a mature manner can also enhance your application.

Ultimately, being observant and asking questions will help you further your understanding of what is required in being a dentist. At the end of each of your placements, you should ask yourself whether this is still a career path that you wish to pursue. If there are any aspects of the work that you dislike, ask yourself whether these would put you off becoming a dentist.

Case study: Maisie Shay, second-year dentistry student

'Dentistry appealed to me primarily because I wanted to pursue a lifelong, vocational career. I liked the fact that dentistry is practical and involves dealing with people regularly, but also that it presents a number of business opportunities.

'When conducting research into possible careers, I undertook a number of work experience placements to ensure that dentistry was the right route for me. My placements involved shadowing dentists in a hospital orthodontics department, in a hospital maxillofacial department, in a private dental practice and in an NHS dental practice. These placements highlighted the wide range of opportunities available as a dentist, with numerous specialities and career routes available upon graduation. I really enjoyed the fast-paced, ever-changing nature of the hospital environments; but in a private practice, the dentist was able to spend more time with patients, allowing more of a relationship to form. The experiences were all very different, but the overarching takeaway was that dentistry is tough and requires continual adaptation and development of skills.

'I was successful in my application to study dentistry at Cardiff University while studying A levels in Biology, Chemistry and Religious Studies, but unfortunately I fell short of my grades on results day. Thankfully, as Cardiff was my first-choice university, they held my place for a year to give me the opportunity to achieve my grades, without having to repeat the UCAT or interviews, and I gained entry the following year. When working on my application, I found that there were many useful online resources, such as students who have previously gone through the process giving their insights and tips. Listening to these insights was invaluable. I also found that attending a UCAT course was beneficial as it provided plenty of timed practice and resources.

'I am now in my second year at Cardiff. The course has been very demanding, with a lot of contact hours and assessments (though much of the content covered in the first year was similar to or an extension of the material covered within A level Biology). We also had lectures based in the dental hospital once a week covering content such as professionalism, which were really insightful and useful in preparing us for patient contact. We also did a lot of relevant practical work to hone these skills.

'I enjoy the practical elements of the course, and at Cardiff we are lucky to have the opportunity to carry out dissections on full body cadavers, which gives you a fundamental knowledge of the anatomy of the face and neck and sets you up for future lectures.

'I also enjoy the social elements: as the course has a small cohort, you get to know everyone quite well, which helps with the transition from school to university. However, the course is very content heavy, so there are times where you have to think about your time management and choose whether to socialise or do your work, which was difficult when settling into first year. It is also very different from A level study in that you have to take a very proactive, independent approach and be strict with yourself to keep on top of the heavy workload, as there is no one making sure that you are.

There were also points in first year where the content felt somewhat irrelevant to dentistry, which was frustrating at times, but it is essential to have a solid grounding before moving on to more technical material.

'Since the Covid-19 pandemic hit, the majority of our lectures have moved online. This hasn't been a hindrance as it means that you can commit the time you need to each lecture to ensure that you understand the content thoroughly; but it does mean that your days are less structured, as many are pre-recorded and, without clear organisation, it would be very easy to fall behind. Practice with the phantom head and in-person clinical skills have been put on hold for now. This has been unavoidable but disappointing, though this time should be made up when it is safe to do so.

'In the future, I am confident that my hard work will pay off, though at the moment, I am still uncertain which speciality I will pursue. I also hope to run my own practice one day.'

The importance of voluntary work

In addition to undertaking work experience directly related to dentistry, it is also essential to show evidence or experience of any voluntary work that you have undertaken. The most useful voluntary work to undertake would be in a care-based environment, for example, a hospital, a children's hospice or a nursing home. Second best would be voluntary work in settings such as schools, youth clubs and community groups. Still useful, but least desirable would be time spent in a charity shop. Most charitable organisations are always eager to recruit volunteers to help out, so these kinds of experience are usually far easier to arrange than a placement in a dental surgery.

The point of carrying out voluntary work is to demonstrate the caring side of your personality and also develop your ability to deal with people. If you have been able to put together a well-developed portfolio of experience, it will go a long way to demonstrate to admissions tutors that you are really devoted to working with and helping people. It will also help to develop your understanding of the wider world and other clinical environments and so ultimately strengthen your application.

Making the most of your work experience and voluntary work

The notebook that you record the details of your experiences in will quickly become a personal diary of what you have completed, and this will be an invaluable resource when it comes to writing a personal statement. Should you be offered an interview, it is extremely likely that you will be asked questions about the experiences you have shared in your statement, so including details you have recorded will give you a chance to talk about a topic you are at ease with. Similarly, many dental schools will request further information about your work experience – including reflection on what you have learned – so having easy access to this information will be very beneficial.

Start by noting down the dates and duration of each of your placements; this is a vital element that will need to be included in your personal statement to show that you have not just done the minimum amount of experience to be considered. Often, students that have done months and months of work experience will undersell themselves by not giving this level of detail.

You should also make sure you note down descriptions of what you have done or seen each day; try to remember names of specific treatments or procedures that you have seen and remember to ask if you don't know the technical name of a procedure or a piece of equipment. This will allow you to build an understanding of some of the technical terminology used in the profession and help you to build an understanding of the day-to-day responsibilities of a dentist.

Finally, the most important thing for you to do is to carry out deep reflection on the time you have spent undertaking work experience and voluntary placements. It is vital that you go beyond simple descriptions of what you have seen and delve more into what stood out to you and what your thoughts and feelings were, as this will demonstrate that you really engaged with what you saw. If you are not able to do this successfully in a personal statement and at interview, you are much less likely to come across well.

Case study: Shyam Patel, fifth-year dentistry student

'When considering what I wanted to do as a career, I knew that I would find an office-based job boring. Dentistry appealed to me because it requires a unique skillset involving carrying out practical work to a high technical degree alongside helping patients, which I knew I would find to be very satisfying. I also wanted to be the first doctor in my family and make them proud! I also considered medicine for this reason, but when comparing the two through research and work experience, I found I preferred dentistry as it allowed for greater continuity with patients and the development of relationships.

'I conducted my work experience in a local, family-run practice. It was an insightful experience, which showed me how a dentist can do a great deal for a wide range of patients with varying problems. I learned that dentistry has developed rapidly over the last few decades, especially with the changes to the UDA (Units of Dental Activity), and that it is likely to keep developing in the future. Perhaps most importantly, I learned that being a dentist is certainly not an easy job – it requires a great deal of technical skill and you must be able to carry out tasks in a coordinated manner while dealing directly with people.

'My experience at A level was challenging as my sixth form tried to prevent me from studying the second year of A level Chemistry. I was fortunately able to transfer to a more supportive school where I achieved good A level grades in Biology, Chemistry and Psychology. I also performed well on the UCAT exam and secured an interview and an offer from the University of Plymouth, where I am now in my final year.

'Studying dentistry has been the best decision of my life, and I have loved every minute of it. The first two years of the course at Plymouth was very theoretical, with a large focus on bioscience and anatomy. Further into the course, there was a more clinical focus, which is the component that I enjoyed the most. This early clinical exposure at Plymouth put me in a good place in terms of patient management and confidence in providing treatment. A typical day in the clinic is spent at a chair with my clinical partner, taking turns as the dentist with the other acting as the nurse. We started clinical practice in the final term of Year 1, where we saw patients once a week. In Years 2 and 3, this increased to twice a week, and prior to the lockdown brought about by Covid-19, we saw patients three times a week in Year 4. While we have continued to have clinical contact in Year 5, it is currently restricted to non-aerosol generating procedures other than at allocated times.

'The global Covid-19 pandemic has affected dentistry a great deal. The dental handpiece operates at 200–400k RPM and uses a water spray to prevent it getting too hot. This generates the most aerosols of any profession, which ultimately puts dental teams at significant risk. However, strict guidelines have been introduced which affects the way we treat patients; there is more PPE and a fallow time (time to air a room out after a procedure) between patients, both of which make it harder and more time-consuming to treat patients. Hopefully, things will change in the future.

'There are many aspects I have enjoyed about the course. Many patients locally have been deprived of regular dental care, so they come into the dental school requiring a lot of work. There is a great sense of satisfaction in providing a service for people in need.

Dentistry can be a very demanding course, but the rewards often override this and make the pressure easier to manage.

'I have really enjoyed living in the South-west, and in Year 4 I lived in Cornwall and treated patients in Truro, which was great as some of the best beaches in the UK were only a short drive away.

'In ten years' time, I hope to be a successful dentist with my own mixed private and NHS practice. The Bachelor of Dental Surgery (BDS) is a baseline for a dentist, and there is plenty of room for professional development and further education. I hope to continue my studies in oral surgery and implantology in the future.

'My advice for prospective dental students is: don't give up. If you are serious about being a dentist, then keep pursuing it, regardless of the approach that you have to take. This might involve studying a broad undergraduate degree, such as biomedical science, or studying dentistry abroad or studying dental hygiene (a three-year course that allows you to learn some of the scope of a dentist but without being able to carry out advanced treatment).'

Work experience and voluntary work during the pandemic

At the time of writing, the coronavirus pandemic continued to disrupt our daily lives, and therefore impact a student's ability to acquire work experience, especially in the field of dentistry. Dental departments were limiting the number of non-frontline staff for safety reasons, making it even more difficult to gain access to these highly sought-after positions, and the number of procedures that could be conducted was also limited, meaning the scope for observation was reduced. As such, most dental schools recognised that getting a set amount of work experience could be problematic. If you are unable to undertake a work experience placement in a dentistry setting because of Covid-19 restrictions, contact the relevant university admissions department to clarify that they will still consider your application, and they should be sympathetic given the gravity of the situation.

The Dental Schools Council issued a statement relating to work experience requirements during the Covid-19 pandemic, which assures students applying to study dentistry that the disruption brought about by the pandemic will be taken into account. This statement can be read at www.dentalschoolscouncil.ac.uk/news/dsc-releases-advice-on-gaining-experience-to-study-dentistry-during-the-covid-19-pandemic.

That being said, dentistry school admissions officers will still be looking for an in-depth understanding of the dentistry profession, including what the career entails and the values and skills required to be a dentist, so you will need to be creative in your approach to gaining this understanding. As well as talking to dentists and dentistry students, there are numerous online resources that will assist you in obtaining this knowledge. At the time of writing, there were no virtual dentistry work experience opportunities, but as the profession adapts to the pandemic these might well become available.

There are things that you can do to support your application in the midst of a pandemic:

- **Keep an eye on the news.** Throughout the pandemic, the media has covered many aspects from presenting facts and figures to giving an insight into how healthcare workers have been impacted. Some media sources will put a political spin on their stories, so you will need to read from a variety of sources to get a balanced view.
- **Voluntary work.** As with work experience, voluntary work within healthcare settings is likely to be disrupted, but the pandemic has brought about other voluntary opportunities that are worth exploring. The purpose of voluntary work is to gain an insight into care work, as well as learning about your own skills and attributes. Providing it is safe for you to do so, you could explore whether any local community groups require support, or perhaps even online opportunities, such as support groups. Nextdoor (https://nextdoor. co.uk) and Do It (https://do-it.org) are organisations that coordinate voluntary work.
- **Independent learning.** Practising dentistry involves a life-long commitment to learning, so taking it upon yourself to learn something medicine-related can demonstrate that you are willing to do this. This can involve reading around topics of interest online, listening to podcasts or watching relevant TED Talks. You could also complete an online course, such as those provided by FutureLearn (www.futurelearn.com), which usually run over a period of a few weeks. A popular course on this platform is 'Discover Dentistry', organised by the University of Sheffield, which provides an excellent insight into the profession.
- **Online resources and social media.** Many students and dentists present their life journeys through social media platforms such as YouTube and Instagram, as well as through blogs. While informal, these can still provide a useful insight into the realities of dentistry as a career.

University admission officers will also want to see that you understand the qualities required to succeed as a dentist, such as effective communication and being able to interact with a wide range of people. It would therefore be useful to consider the NHS Constitution, the details of which can be found here: www.gov.uk/government/publications/the-nhs-constitution-for-england/the-nhs-constitution-for-england.

3 | Choosing your course

To gain a place at dental school, you have to submit a UCAS application. However, before you do so it is essential that you have thoroughly researched the application process, entrance requirements and the demands of dentistry as a profession. Most people have little understanding of the tasks and challenges that a dentist faces on a day-to-day basis and the career pathways available after graduation. It is therefore vital that you are aware both of what being a dentist entails and of the details of the application process before you consider applying to study dentistry. This will ultimately mean that whatever choice you make it will be a well-informed one.

Choice of school

Once you have completed your work experience and are sure that you want to be a dentist, you need to thoroughly research your choice of dental school.

There are various factors that you should take into account:

- the structure of the course and teaching styles employed
- the academic requirements needed to gain entry to the course
- whether the dental school requires you to sit the UCAT or BMAT
- the location and type of university
- whether the dental school is part of a large university or is a stand-alone medical and dental school.

The majority of information about each university and course can be found on the UCAS website (www.ucas.com) and the individual university websites, so it is well worth spending some time looking here. If you cannot find the answers you need, feel free to call, email, or attend the university open day with any questions relating to admissions or to the course itself. In Chapter 11, there is a list of major dental organisations in the UK that you can contact for further information, and a list of the dental schools and their contact details. What you must remember is that information on websites is always changing, so if you're in doubt it is always best to call the university and speak to someone to get the most up-to-date information.

Remember that when researching different dental courses (and when you come to apply via UCAS), it is vital to make sure that you choose the right course and course code. There are a number of slight variations in the course title and code depending on the type and duration of the course. The five-year undergraduate dentistry course will have the UCAS code A200, A205 or A206, so check this as part of your research.

Apart from talking to current or former dental students or careers advisers, there are a number of other sources of information that will help you in making your choice. There are various independent league tables of dental schools, ranked by a total score that combines several assessment categories, including teaching scores, student–staff ratios and job prospects. For instance, the *Complete University Guide* (www. thecompleteuniversityguide.co.uk) 2019 rankings looked like this:

Table 2 *Complete University Guide* dental school rankings

Rank	University
1st	University of Glasgow
2nd	University of Dundee
3rd	Queen Mary, University of London
4th	Newcastle University
5th	Cardiff University
6th	University of Bristol
7th	University of Sheffield
8th	University of Manchester
9th	King's College London
10th	University of Birmingham
11th	Queen's University Belfast
12th	University of Leeds
13th	University of Aberdeen
14th	University of Liverpool
15th	University of Central Lancashire
16th	University of Plymouth

Source: www.thecompleteuniversityguide.co.uk/league-tables/rankings?s=dentistry
Reprinted with kind permission from the *Complete University Guide*

Of course, there is no such thing as a bad dental school in the UK, and league tables tell you only a small part of the whole story. They are based on a range of variables and this is why there can be discrepancies between different websites. Remember that league tables are only a guide – they are no substitute for visiting the dental schools, looking at the course content in detail and speaking to those involved with the course.

Open days

As well as researching dental schools online, you can also learn a great deal about them by visiting on open days. Information about open days can be obtained from university websites, or websites such as www. opendays.com. By attending an organised open day, you will be able to see the departments in which you could be studying and meet current academic staff and students, who will be able to answer any questions that you might have. You can also get a feel for the university – you could be spending the next five years of your life there, so it is important that you feel comfortable in that environment. If you don't, you might struggle to see the course through, irrespective of your academic achievements.

If you are planning on attending an open day, it is important that you ensure that you book onto any relevant talks to give yourself the best possible chance of obtaining the information that you need.

If you are unable to attend an organised open day, you should contact the university and ascertain whether there are any other opportunities to visit the department. In many cases, there will be someone who is able to meet you and give you a brief tour. If this is not possible, you can still visit on an informal basis to have a look around the university and see whether you like it, though you may not be able to visit the dental school itself.

Virtual Open Days

In light of the coronavirus pandemic, many universities have converted their open days into virtual events that are conducted wholly online in order to protect the health of prospective students. A virtual open day is different to visiting a campus in person, but it is still an excellent opportunity to see what a university has to offer and get an insight into a place where you might be studying. While some universities will look to reinstate face-to-face open days in the coming months, virtual open days will persist as they have many benefits.

As you won't have to factor in travel to the universities, you can attend more open days than you might have initially intended. This might open up more doors for you in terms of your dental school options.

Virtual open days have differing formats depending on the university, but typically provide an opportunity to take virtual tours, attend online webinars and talk to current students, lecturers and admissions officers, allowing you to ask any questions that you might have.

Non-academic considerations

When attending a university open day, there are a number of non-academic points to consider that will give you a better idea of whether the course is for you or not. You should start by considering the university itself – think about the following points:

- location of the university and distance from home: some students prefer to live at home or be very close to home, while others like to get as far away as possible
- campus or city university: again, students seem to have strong preferences about the type of university they study at; some prefer to be in the middle of a big city while others like to be situated on a rural campus, and visiting the university is the only way to get a true feel for its character
- social and sporting facilities: most universities have good sporting facilities, but there will naturally be variation in the standard and range of what is available and how far students will have to travel to access these facilities
- accommodation, location and cost: whether the university is a campus or city university will usually have an impact on the location of the accommodation. Usually campus universities will have accommodation on campus or very close by, while city universities will often have it spread out across a wider area. This can have a big impact on the amount of time you spend each day travelling to and from lectures. The quality of accommodation can also vary widely between universities, so it is worth researching the range of different rooms available rather than just the high-end rooms that you are likely to be shown on an open day
- size of the university and student population: although not a major factor for most students, some like the idea of being part of a very large student group, while others prefer smaller universities with a more intimate community.

When you take time to visit a university you will automatically get a feel for these points. From this you should consider whether it is the sort of place where you would like to study. It is not uncommon for students to think they would like to go to a particular university and then totally change their mind about it after taking the time to visit.

Academic requirements

In addition to the grades they require at A level, most dental schools have specific GCSE requirements too. Currently, GCSE requirements vary widely from dental school to dental school, but having at least five 7/8 or A/A* grades, with at least 7/A grades in science subjects, English language and mathematics will be a significant advantage. In recent years, there have been a number of dental schools that have relaxed their admissions policies in terms of GCSE requirements; however, it still remains a considerable advantage to significantly exceed the minimum requirements they ask for. If your grades fall below the GCSE requirements set for a particular dentistry course, there is little or no point in applying to that particular university; university admissions tutors often comment on how many applicants they immediately reject because they do not meet the published requirements. If you have genuine extenuating circumstances that explain why you have underachieved (due to illness, family circumstances, etc.), you will need to contact the university to enquire whether they will take this into consideration. In all cases, it is expected that your referee will include in your reference details of the extenuating circumstances that you faced.

Since the A level reform, AS grades now act as standalone qualifications. If you have completed AS level examinations, these are likely to be taken into account by the admissions tutors reviewing your application. As such, if it is your school's policy for you to sit these exams in year 12, it is important that you take them seriously.

The A level requirements vary between dental schools, but most ask for Chemistry and Biology at A level alongside a third A level. In recent years, some universities have relaxed their stance on these requirements: Plymouth now requires Biology at A level, plus a second science from Chemistry, Physics, Maths or Psychology; Queen Mary, University of London now asks for Biology or Chemistry, plus one other science from Biology, Chemistry, Physics or Maths; and King's College London asks for Biology or Chemistry, plus one other science from Biology, Chemistry, Physics, Maths or Psychology. While these options make it possible to pursue dentistry without one of Biology or Chemistry, your options will be rather limited, so studying both would give you the best possible chance.

In the past, a number of dental schools accepted A level students who had not achieved the required grades the first time. Unfortunately, due to the competitive nature of dentistry courses, it can be more challenging to gain access to dentistry courses as a retake student, though it is not impossible. There are a few courses that will still consider retake applications, but some will have certain criteria attached. Take the University of Manchester, for example, where retake students can apply, but only if they have already achieved BBB at A level in the first sitting. If you are in a position where you want to pursue dentistry but need to retake your A level exams, you will need to conduct careful research into your options to ensure that each of your UCAS choices is carefully selected to give you the best possible chance.

Table 3 (opposite) shows which dental schools consider students who have not achieved the minimum grades at their first attempt. If there

Table 3 Dental school admissions policies – 2020/21

University	Standard offer	GCSE requirements	Retakes considered?	Retake offer	A level subject requirements	UCAT policy
Queen's Belfast (A200)	AAA	Minimum 4/C in GCSE Mathematics and English if not offered at AS/A level. GCSE performance in the best 9 subjects will be scored with 4 points awarded for a 9/A* and 3 for an 8/7/A. Points are not awarded for 6/B and 5/C.	Yes – if applied to Queen's at first attempt, held an offer as their first choice and achieved AAB at first sitting.	–	Biology/Human Biology and Chemistry	Required
Birmingham (A200)	AAA	Chemistry and Biology at 9/A*. 7/A in Maths and English Language or Literature.	No, for both GCSE and A level.	–	Chemistry and Biology	Required
Bristol (A206)	AAA (AAC/ABB if certain contextual criteria are considered)	7/A in GCSE Mathematics and 4/C in GCSE English or equivalent.	Yes, both GCSE and A level. A maximum of one resit is allowed in any one subject.	–	Chemistry and one of Biology, Physics or Mathematics	Required
Cardiff (A200)	AAA	6/B in English Language. Six GCSEs, including 7/A in sciences.	No, unless you have held a conditional firm offer in the previous year and not met the conditions of that offer.	–	Biology and Chemistry at grade A (Critical Thinking and General Studies are excluded)	Required
Dundee (A200)	AAA	Biology and Chemistry to at least GCSE grade 7/AB, Maths and another subject to at least grade 6/B.	No	–	Chemistry and another science (Biology is recommended, General Studies is not accepted)	Required

Table 3 Continued

University	Standard offer	GCSE requirements	Retakes considered?	Retake offer	A level subject requirements	UCAT policy
Glasgow (A200)	AAA	Six subjects at 7/A, must include Mathematics and/or Physics. English Language or Literature at 6/B.	No	–	Biology and Chemistry	Required
King's (A205)	A*AA + B at AS	At least 6/B in English Language and Mathematics.	No	–	Biology or Chemistry, plus one from Biology, Chemistry, Physics, Maths or Psychology	Required
Leeds (A200)	AAA	Six at 6/B or above, including Chemistry, Biology (or Dual Science), plus English and Mathematics.	Yes	AAA	Biology and Chemistry	Not required, but BMAT is
Liverpool (A200)	AAA	Minimum of eight, with a minimum of five 7/As and three 6/Bs. Mathematics, English Language and Science at 6/B or above.	No	–	Biology and Chemistry	Required
Manchester (A206)	AAA	Five at 8/A* or 7/A with 6/B or above in English Language, Mathematics and two science subjects.	Yes – minimum BBB at first sitting.	A*AA with A* in either Biology or Chemistry	Biology and Chemistry	Required

Table 3 Continued

Newcastle (A206)	AAA	No specific requirements.	No	–	Biology and Chemistry	Required
Plymouth (A206)	A*AA – AAB (contextual offer)	Seven at 9–4/A–C, including English Language, Mathematics and either Single and Additional Science or Biology and Chemistry.	Yes – if achieved ABB at first sitting	A*AA–AAA	Biology and one from Chemistry, Mathematics, Physics and Psychology	Required
Queen Mary (A200)	A*AA	Minimum three 7/As and three 6/Bs, to include Biology, Chemistry, English Language and Mathematics; the Science Double Award may substitute any individual science.	No	–	Biology or Chemistry and one other science (Chemistry, Biology, Physics or Mathematics)	Required
Sheffield (A200)	AAA	Six at 7/A, including Mathematics, English Language and Science.	Yes	AAA	Biology and Chemistry	Required

All information taken from www.ucas.com and from individual university websites.

have been genuine extenuating circumstances that have caused you to underachieve and you have evidence of this, then it is worth talking to each university to see if they will consider your application, as there can be some leeway here in terms of being considered as a retake student. However, the prevailing conditions are that an increasing number of universities either don't consider extenuating circumstances or require the circumstances to have been reported to the examination boards at the time that the examinations were taken.

Another issue to be considered is the requirement to have an A* grade at A level. For entry in 2021, Queen Mary, University of London and King's College London both stated that a typical offer includes an A*. For students who are retaking their A levels, universities (including the University of Manchester and Plymouth University) might also include an A* as part of their offer.

The impact of Covid-19 on dental school places

Results day in August 2020 was an unpleasant time for many aspiring dentists. Students in this cohort had their exams cancelled and were instead awarded calculated grades based on an Ofqual-derived algorithm. Many students found themselves with much lower grades than they had anticipated, which led to them losing their hard-earned dental school places. As with any other year, dental schools were then tasked with filling places in the days following results day. Despite promising that there would be no U-turn on results, the Government ultimately decided that they would instead award the highest grade out of the calculated grade, Centre Assessed Grade (CAG) – i.e. the grade the school submitted for them – and the moderated grade awarded by Ofqual or the grade achieved in an October resit exam. With CAGs being awarded, there were many more students who had met the conditions of their offers than places available. As such, this meant that many students who had met the conditions of their offer were not guaranteed a place for 2020 entry.

To assist with the placement of successful students, the Department for Education agreed to lift the cap on dental school places and provided confirmation of additional funding to support both university and clinical placements. While this was a positive move, it left many questions regarding placements for 2021, as successful candidates had their places deferred and the 2021 applicant cohort have had their sixth-form studies significantly disrupted by Covid-19. Despite the increased intake for 2020 and a number of places being deferred for 2021, dental schools intend to recruit in line with their normal numbers for 2021 entry at the time of writing, with pressure on the Department for Education to provide additional places for a second year in a row.

The UCAS Tariff

The UCAS tariff system allocates a certain number of points for each qualification achieved. This system allows direct comparison of standards achieved in different qualifications, such as the International Baccalaureate and Scottish Highers, but is mainly used as a tool for universities to report data to the government.

It is worth keeping the details of the tariff in mind if you need to refer to it, but remember that currently all dental offers are made in terms of grades rather than UCAS Tariff points. The Tariff is as follows:

A level grades	UCAS Tariff points
A*	56
A	48
B	40
C	32
D	24
E	16

Other qualifications

If you are not studying A levels, you should check with each dental school about their requirements. The list below offers a rough indication of what they might ask for in a selection of qualifications commonly offered as an alternative to A level study.

- **Scottish Highers:** AAABB–AAAAA at Higher level and two or three subjects at Advanced Higher. Higher level Chemistry and Biology are usually required. Most universities require two to three Advanced Highers, usually including Chemistry and Biology at grades AA/AAA.
- **International Baccalaureate:** 6, 6, 6 to 6, 6, 7 and 32–38 points overall. Chemistry and biology should be usually taken at Higher level.
- **Cambridge Pre-U:** most universities will accept Cambridge Pre-U qualifications with D3, D3, M3/D3 in the principal subjects. Biology and Chemistry will usually be required as principal subjects.
- **BTEC National Diploma:** a few universities are happy to accept this with three Distinctions, but usually only when offered alongside some A level subjects such as Chemistry and Biology. Once again, it is best to contact the individual universities to discuss their entry requirements.

You will need to check with each university about its specific entry requirements as there is always some variation in their demands. If you have studied qualifications that are not listed here, then you should also check their suitability directly with the university.

Non-dental choices

Although you can apply to a total of five institutions through UCAS, you may apply to only *four* dental schools. So, what should you do with the final slot? Applying for an alternative, non-dental course will not jeopardise your dentistry application in any way, but the fifth choice is still worthy of careful consideration for a number of reasons. There are two main options regarding the fifth choice.

Do not include a fifth choice

If you are truly committed to becoming a dentist, you need to consider whether you would realistically accept the course you chose to include as a fifth choice. If you know that you would not consider that course and would prefer to reapply for dentistry, it may be in your best interests to leave the final choice blank. If you were then unfortunate enough to not secure a place to study dentistry, you could spend a year developing your application in order to boost your chances the following year.

Carefully consider an alternative course

You might choose to include a non-dental choice on your form if you are not prepared to wait for a year if your application is unsuccessful, or if you are happy to enter a dentistry course as a graduate.

Trying to combine two different subjects in your personal statements is a recipe for disaster. Although admissions tutors cannot see which other courses you have applied for on your UCAS application, it may be obvious to both departments that you are not really committed to either course. This would be especially apparent if you were including a completely unrelated subject as your fifth choice. As such, do not try to combine two subjects in your personal statement – simply stick to dentistry.

If there is a course that you would genuinely consider studying in place of dentistry, or perhaps you are already reapplying and just want to go to university next academic year regardless of the course, there are ways of applying to two separate courses.

If you do intend to include a fifth choice, then you may need to contact the university in question to ascertain whether or not they will consider this application. Many universities will happily consider this option once you have contacted them to explain why your personal statement does not match up with the course, but some may request an additional personal statement. In this case, be prepared to deliver a second personal statement outlining why you are committed to studying that course if you are to successfully acquire a place. Such requests are becoming especially common where students choose other vocational degrees, such as pharmacy or optometry, as their back-up choices.

Many students also pursue the option of undertaking a first degree in a related subject – such as biomedical materials science or biochemistry – which they then utilise as a platform to gain access onto dentistry as a second degree. Whether or not to consider a BSc in lieu of a dentistry degree is a tricky question, and ultimately, it can be answered by no one other than you. There are several pros and cons worth considering.

Pros

- Dentistry is a life-long commitment, so two to three years of additional study should not worry you. Becoming a good dentist is a journey, not a target.
- Applying as a graduate certainly makes your dental school application stronger as you have matured as an individual and academically.
- Having a BSc as well as a dental degree may enhance your chances of getting the job you desire (and is a reason why many dental students intercalate).
- Studying a first degree will give you time to mature as a person. You will become acquainted with the demands of university life and develop your skills in independent study. Many students who take this approach find that by the time they reach dental school, they are more comfortable with the workload and can approach the study of dentistry with greater confidence.

Cons

- You might spend a whole three years on a course you never really wanted to study. Studying a subject at degree level is an enormous commitment, and if you are not entirely motivated by the content, it can be a very trying time.
- Three years of study will add additional cost and time before actually getting into dental school.
- Entry to dental school after graduating is not guaranteed. Although some BSc courses do offer a pathway to dental school, these places are often only available to the highest achievers and can therefore be just as competitive as applying directly to study dentistry.
- If admitted to undergraduate dental school only, you will still have to study for five more years.
- You might lose focus on dentistry if you study something else first.
- You may not get the student funding and help towards fees, compared with if you go straight after A levels.

Case study: Dr Khaleda Shah, University of Liverpool graduate

'Before studying dentistry, I completed an undergraduate degree in medical science at the University of Birmingham. After graduating, I wasn't entirely sure what I wanted to do as a career, but I got a job in medical sales and was very successful. While the financial benefits were good, it wasn't a particularly rewarding role so I reflected on what I would like to do. I had worked as a carer previously and really enjoyed patient interaction, so did some research into healthcare roles and work experience and decided to apply to study dentistry. I studied graduate-entry dentistry at the University of Liverpool. This was a challenging time as I had to work several part-time jobs to support myself, but it was definitely worth it.

'I am currently completing my foundation training which is compulsory if you want to work for the NHS. I am currently training in "maxfax" in a hospital, specialising in oral surgery. This has been a really rewarding role as you can see the effects of giving patients back their confidence, and there is significant scope for learning beyond what you may come across in a general dental practice. However, there are some challenging aspects to the role, and these include patients being quite difficult and demanding, wanting instant fixes rather than working towards what they are looking to achieve.

'At the moment, Covid-19 is really disrupting the way that things would usually be done, especially as we are working in the mouth and would typically be using aerosol-generating procedures. Having to adapt has been a steep learning curve! Dentistry during the pandemic has been slow, and patients have understandably been frustrated at not getting the treatment that they want or need in as timely a manner as they might be used to. The system that was put in place has struggled to cope with patient demands, but we are slowly getting back in control.

'My advice to aspiring dentists and dental students would be to make sure that you have something else in your life. Dentistry can be stressful, and while it's good to be committed and motivated, it shouldn't be your only focus, as you will need something else that you can do to unwind.'

4| The UCAS application

Navigating your way through the UCAS application process can be a daunting process at times. This chapter breaks the process down in order to help you understand each of the stages.

UCAS Apply

When you apply for UK universities, you do so using the UCAS Apply system. The online UCAS form is accessed through the UCAS website (www.ucas.com). You register online either through your school or college, or as a private individual. Some of the information that you provide on the form is factual, such as where you live, where you have studied, what academic qualifications you have, details of examinations that you are going to take, and which university courses you are applying for. Other sections, such as the personal statement and reference, allow more expansive information to be communicated. The sections of the UCAS form are as follows:

- **Personal Details:** this includes all of your basic personal information as well as contact details and details of criminal convictions and any special educational needs.
- **Additional Information:** in this section, you enter details of your ethnicity, parental occupations and details of any activities that you have completed in preparation for higher education.
- **Student Finance:** this section asks about your intention to apply for student finance and if you wish your details to be shared automatically with the student finance organisations.
- **Choices:** this is where you enter your course choices.
- **Education:** this section is used to provide details of all of the schools and colleges you have attended (not including primary school) and the details of the qualifications you have received there.
- **Employment:** in this section, include details of any paid employment.
- **Personal Statement:** this is where you put your personal statement once it is completed.
- **Reference and Predicted Grades:** finally, this is where your academic referee enters their reference about you and the grades you have been predicted for each subject.

Once your form is complete, it is accessed by the person who will write your reference; they then check your form, add the reference and predicted grades and send it to UCAS. Remember that when you have completed your form and pressed 'send', the form does not go straight to UCAS, but is instead sent to the person who oversees the UCAS process at your school or college. This means that your form can be returned to you at this point if there are any mistakes that need correcting. If you register as a private individual, a request for your reference will be sent to the person you have nominated as your referee. You will only be able to send your form to UCAS once this has been completed, so make contact with your chosen referee early, and remain in communication with them, to ensure there are no delays.

Once your application has been submitted, you can keep track of the responses from the universities using UCAS Track.

When to submit your UCAS application

The closing date for receipt of the application by UCAS is 15 October. Remember that this is the deadline by which the form is required to be submitted to UCAS and so your school or college will most likely have an earlier deadline so it can check your application, get your reference written and send it off to UCAS. This will probably be around two weeks earlier, though this will vary depending on your school. Late applications are accepted by UCAS, but the dental schools are not obliged to consider them; because of the pressure on places, it is unlikely that late applications will be considered. You can submit your application at any time between the beginning of September and 15 October. As long as you don't miss the October deadline, your application will receive the same treatment, regardless of when it is submitted. However, in terms of your own peace of mind, it is always recommended to submit as early as you can.

The safest bet for getting your application completed and sent as soon as possible is to make a start on it in the first year of your A levels. Start researching the different universities and the different courses as soon as possible and then begin writing your personal statement and get feedback on it. Ultimately, you want to be in a position where you have a final draft of your personal statement and all of your choices sorted by the beginning of September in your final year of A levels.

The reference

As well as your GCSE results, personal statement and predicted grades, the admissions team will take into account your academic reference. This is where a relevant teacher – perhaps your headteacher, form tutor or head of sixth form – writes about your academic potential and personal attributes. The referee is expected to be as honest as possible, and to try to accurately assess your character and potential. You may believe that you have all of the qualities – academic and personal – necessary in a dentist, but unless you have demonstrated these to your teachers, they may not be able to support your application.

Ideally, your efforts to impress them will have begun at the start of the sixth form (or preferably before this); you will have become involved in school activities, while at the same time working hard on your A level subjects and developing strong interpersonal skills, demonstrated by your interactions with staff and students. If you do not feel as though you have done this, don't worry, because it is never too late. Some people mature later than others, so if this does not sound like you, start to make efforts to get involved in the wider life of your school or college, as this will help provide evidence for the people who will contribute to your reference.

As part of the reference, your referee will need to predict the grades that you are likely to achieve. As Table 3 in Chapter 3 (see pages 39–41) shows, the most likely minimum requirement for entry is AAA, although some dental schools indicate that they may include an A* as part of the offer. If your predicted grades are lower than this, it is unlikely that you will be considered. Talk to your teachers and find out whether you are on target for these grades. If not, you need to do one or all of the following:

- work harder or more effectively, and make sure that your teachers notice that you are doing so
- get some extra help either at school or outside if possible
- communicate with dental schools to see whether they are likely to make you an offer with the grades you have been predicted
- delay submitting your UCAS application until you have your A level results.

UCAT

All but one of the UK dental schools (Leeds) now require applicants to sit the pre-admissions test known as the UCAT (the University Clinical Aptitude Test) before they apply. This test helps dental school admissions teams to make an informed choice between the highest performing candidates for undergraduate dental study. It is designed to ensure that students have the mental capabilities, attitude and professional conduct required for a career in the dental field. It is not a test of your curriculum knowledge or any scientific background. The UCAT tests thought processes and as such cannot be revised for, though it is possible to prepare yourself in order to boost your overall attainment.

The UCAT is a computer-based test, and this aspect should not be underestimated as your eyes will get very tired after staring at a computer screen for two hours. It is therefore necessary to ensure that at least some of your preparation is done online.

Students have the option of completing the test at an official Pearson VUE test centre or at home (UCAT Online) using Pearson VUE's online proctoring service. Careful consideration should be given as to where you sit the test. The home option was brought in to ensure that the UCAT was accessible to all students, despite the ongoing challenges that the Covid-19 pandemic presents.

If completing your test at a centre, the setting will be unfamiliar, but the more formal testing environment may reduce distractions and aid concentration, and also minimises the possibility of technical failure. Test centres can be found in many locations worldwide, so it is worthwhile identifying which test centres are local to you. If there is a problem with your attending any of these centres, consult the UCAT website (www. ucat.ac.uk).

Sitting the test at home gives you greater flexibility in terms of choosing a test date, and it could minimise the stress of travelling to an unfamiliar test centre. You may be more comfortable sitting your test at home, but consider whether or not you will be distracted, whether your internet connection is sufficient and whether your device meets the technical requirements (this can be assessed using UCAT's System Test in advance). Similarly, there are a number of ID requirements that must be met to sit the UCAT Online, including identity and workspace verification and live proctoring, which involves using a webcam and microphone. If you are below the age of 18, a parent or guardian must be present when you begin your test.

Registration is typically open between May and September and, in previous years, you have been able to sit the test between early July and early October. The earlier you take it, the better, as you will be able to sit the UCAT with a clear head; you will also have more time to research which universities will consider your overall application, inclusive of the UCAT score. In addition, if you become unwell or are unable to make your booked test for any reason, you have the opportunity to reschedule for a later date. If you book your initial test too late in the cycle, then it is unlikely that there will be local slots available.

Because of the Covid-19 pandemic, there was a shift in registration and testing dates in 2020, with registration opening at the beginning of July and testing starting at the beginning of August and finishing at the beginning of October. Applicants were encouraged to sit the UCAT early due to the pandemic and the uncertainty surrounding the testing situation should the UK find itself in lockdown.

> **Dates**
>
> A list of important dates regarding the UCAT exam can be found at www.ucat.ac.uk. At present, the key dates for 2021 remain uncertain due to the continuing nature of the Covid-19 pandemic. For reference, the key dates for 2020 were:
>
> - registration opens: 1 July 2020
> - testing begins: 3 August 2020
> - registration deadline: 12 noon, 17 September 2020
> - last testing date: 1 October 2020.
>
> *Please check www.ucat.ac.uk for 2021 dates.*

If you have any disabilities or additional needs that require you to have extra time in examinations, it is important that you register for the UCATSEN instead of the regular test. For example, if you require 25% additional time in examinations due to a diagnosis of dyslexia, the UCATSEN will allocate this additional time to each section of the exam. If you require special access arrangements for examinations, then you should directly contact Pearson VUE customer services to discuss these arrangements before you book a test.

There are five separately timed sections to the UCAT. These sections are based on a set of skills that both medical and dental schools believe are vital to be successful as a practitioner.

1. **Verbal reasoning.** Candidates are provided with a piece of text that they have to analyse and answer questions on. This section assesses the ability of the candidate to critically evaluate written information.
2. **Decision making.** This test assesses a candidate's ability to apply logic to reach a decision or conclusion, evaluate arguments and analyse statistical information.
3. **Quantitative reasoning.** This section assesses a candidate's ability to critically evaluate information presented in a numerical form.
4. **Abstract reasoning.** Candidates are presented with a series of shapes that they must interpret and identify patterns within. This section assesses the use of convergent and divergent thinking to infer relationships.
5. **Situational judgement.** This tests candidates' ability to comprehend real-world situations and to identify critical factors and appropriate behaviour in handling them.

The test lasts two hours in total. Those candidates with special educational needs take the UCATSEN and are given the allocated additional time per section.

Table 4 Timings for UCAT/UCATSEN

Section	Items	Standard Test Time	Extra Time/ UCATSEN
Verbal Reasoning	44 items	22 minutes	27.5 minutes
Decision Making	29 items	32 minutes	40 minutes
Quantitative Reasoning	36 items	25 minutes	31.25 minutes
Abstract Reasoning	55 items	14 minutes	17.25 minutes
Situational Judgement	690 items	27 minutes	33.75 minutes
Total time		120 minutes	150 minutes

1. Verbal Reasoning

The Verbal Reasoning test is designed to assess your ability to read and think carefully about information, using comprehension passages to get you to draw specific conclusions from the information presented. The test is based upon the verbal reasoning skills required of dentists to take on board often complex information, to analyse it and then to communicate in simple terms to patients. There are 11 text passages which all have four questions to answer. Some questions will test your comprehension skills by asking you to answer 'true', 'false' or 'can't tell'. In general, if a similar statement can be found in the passage, it is true; if it opposes the information in the text, it is false; and if there is no direct reference to the statement in the passage, we can conclude that we can't tell from the information provided. The other type of question tests your critical response and will look for you to draw a conclusion. You will be presented with an incomplete statement or a question and four response options. You need to pick the most suitable response.

The verbal reasoning section is incredibly challenging, as it requires a rapid pace to get through lengthy passages of text and draw conclusions. In reality, you are unlikely to have much spare time on this section, so it is important to answer each question as you move through, even if it is a guess, rather than wasting time by moving backwards and forwards through questions.

Some candidates prefer to scan-read the passage before reading the questions, as this minimises the time spent reading the questions. Other candidates find this complicated, as it is difficult to remember all of the information in the passage. It may therefore be beneficial to scan read the statement before looking for phrases relating to it in the passage. It is really important that you practise as many questions as possible, as this will allow you to identify particular strategies that work for you for each question type.

2. Decision Making

This test assesses a candidate's ability to apply logic to reach a decision or conclusion, evaluate arguments and analyse statistical information.

A number of skills will be assessed in the decision making element of the UCAT, including:

- deductive reasoning
- evaluating arguments
- statistical reasoning
- figural reasoning.

These skills are assessed through a number of question types:

Logical puzzles

With these questions, you are required to make a deductive inference to arrive at a conclusion. It will involve solving a worded puzzle where some information is given, and the rest you are required to solve. When approaching these questions, you should:

- aim to identify the placement of known facts initially, so that they can be used as a reference for the placement of unknown facts
- eliminate any answers that you know cannot be true
- draw out the information using your whiteboard
- only do the working out that is required – if you do not need to complete the whole puzzle to get the answer, don't waste your time!

Syllogisms

Syllogisms are a form of reasoning where a conclusion is drawn based on a given premise: you are given a statement and asked to draw conclusions based on it. When answering these questions, you should:

- make sure that you have a thorough understanding of the premises given, reading them multiple times if required
- read the conclusions carefully and one by one, so that you can decide whether it is true or false after careful consideration
- avoid making assumptions
- pay attention to the use of qualifying terms.

These questions require a 'drag and drop' response. While it seems straightforward, you should make sure that you spend some time practising this using online practice versions of the test.

Interpreting information

With these questions, information will be presented – the form can vary considerably from passages of text to pie charts – and you must interpret it. You will be expected to draw conclusions based on this information. To increase your chances of getting these questions right, you should:

- try to ignore additional information that is given but is not required
- be prepared to use reasoning skills as opposed to prior knowledge
- where possible, round numbers to solve numerical problems as this will save time calculating
- try not to fall into the trap of basing your answers on the believability of a statement that is made.

Recognising assumptions

In these questions, you will be presented with a number of arguments and you are expected to choose the strongest one. To succeed in these questions, you should:

- ignore your prior beliefs as you must base your responses on the information presented to you
- remember that strong arguments will directly relate to the content in the questions, and this is what you should look out for
- remember assumptions will not be correct, so be careful not to select those as your answer.

Venn diagrams

You will be presented with a Venn diagram and you will be asked to draw conclusions from the information presented within it. You can improve your performance in these questions by:

- revisiting this area of maths and revise it thoroughly
- drawing your own Venn diagram to visualise the answer options.

Probabilistic reasoning

In these questions, you will be given some information containing statistical information and will be required to select the most appropriate response. You should:

- revisit the topic of probability and revise it thoroughly
- eliminate any obviously incorrect statement

3. Quantitative Reasoning

The Quantitative Reasoning test is designed to see if you can solve problems using numerical skills. The test requires you to have good maths skills and knowledge of GCSE level maths. That is not the main point of this test, however; it is more a problem-solving exercise in terms of taking information and manipulating it with calculations and ratios.

As dentists are always using data, it is necessary to test this faculty. From drug calculations to research, applicants need to be able to show they have the ability to cope and can respond to different scenarios.

The data will be presented in a variety of ways, including tables, charts and graphs. Not all of the information provided will be immediately obvious, and it will require your close attention to detail to interpret them. Some data sets may not be presented visually at all, and you will be required to pick out the information from passages of text.

While there is some expectation of mathematical ability, you do not have to be exceptionally good at maths to perform well in the quantitative reasoning section. What is more important is being able to identify the appropriate information in the question and avoid making minor errors through carelessness, which is easily done in the time-pressured environment. In fact, some questions may not require you to do any calculations at all, but rather pick out information from visual data such as graphs and pie charts. Many of the calculations are relatively simple, and can be done by estimating.

A major drawback of the numerical reasoning component of the test is that the calculator is on-screen. Practising using an on-screen calculator as you work through questions in preparation is key for familiarising yourself with the process. While it only takes a few seconds longer than using an ordinary calculator, time is of the essence with this section, so any time that can be saved by carrying out calculations mentally will be incredibly valuable!

Sample questions are provided on the following pages. There are nine sets, each containing four questions, and you will have to choose between five answers. It is a practice-driven section and, as with maths, the more practice you do, the more familiar you will be with answering the questions.

It is worth committing a small proportion of your preparation time to reviewing your knowledge of some key mathematical skills and practising your mental maths so that you are more confident in your approach to more straightforward calculations.

- Being able to convert between percentages and fractions.
- Calculating the area of shapes, e.g. quadrilaterals, triangles and circles.
- Calculating the perimeter of shapes.
- Calculating the circumference of a circle.
- Calculating the volume of an object.
- Calculating percentages.
- Calculating percentage change.

4. Abstract Reasoning

Abstract Reasoning is designed to assess whether you can look at abstract shapes and then identify patterns, while ignoring the irrelevant material to avoid arriving at the wrong conclusion. What this test aims to do is test whether you are able to change your stance, be critical in your evaluations and create a hypothesis through inquiry.

Patients often give dentists numerous symptoms that dentists have to work through to work out what is relevant and what is not in order to arrive at a diagnosis. Dentists therefore have to use their judgement, as patients are not always accurate in the information they provide.

The patterns that you can be presented with will vary considerably, and some patterns will be far more complex than others. The ability to rapidly identify patterns comes easier to some people than others, but the key is to practise: the more patterns you see and become familiar with, the more readily you will be able to identify them. The abstract reasoning section is the fastest on the whole UCAT exam, so preparation is key!

In the UCAT test, you may see one of four items.

- **Type 1:** two sets of shapes labelled 'Set A' and 'Set B'. From a test shape, you need to decide which set the shape belongs to, or neither.
- **Type 2:** From a series of shapes, you need to select the next shape in the series.
- **Type 3:** A statement will be given about a group of shapes and you then need to conclude which shape would complete the statement.
- **Type 4:** Two sets of shapes will be given to you labelled 'Set A' and 'Set B' and you need to decide from four options which belongs to Set A or Set B.

When approaching abstract reasoning questions, the most important aspect is to identify the pattern in each set. The easiest way of doing this is to pick two shapes – it is advisable to choose the most simplistic – and identify what is common about them. Each set will include shapes that are redundant and play no role in the pattern, so you must get used to ignoring these. For some shapes, there will be one common feature, whereas others may have multiple. These can be to do with the number, size, orientation, positioning and colour of the shapes, as well as the shapes themselves.

5. Situational Judgement

The Situational Judgement Test is designed to measure how you deal with real-world situations and whether you can identify critical factors and apply appropriate behaviour in the handling of them. What it is ultimately measuring is the level of integrity and perspective you will bring to the profession and whether you are able to work in a multi-disciplinary team.

The score of the Situational Judgement Test is recorded as a 'band', with band 1 representing the highest score and band 4 representing the lowest. These scores are not included in the UCAT average score but are recorded independently and, as such, are typically used separately by dental schools.

You will be presented with 22 different scenarios and each one will have different actions that you could take, with varying considerations. Typically, these considerations will be in line with maintaining a consistently high level of professionalism, having an understanding of medical ethics and recognising the importance of patient safety. There is no expectation that you will have the procedural knowledge to answer these, but it is worth remembering a few key points.

- Under no circumstances should a dentist, or any other medical professional, carry out any action that may affect the confidence of patients in the profession.
- Problems must be addressed as quickly as possible to reassure the patient.
- Where possible, solutions must be identified and put into place efficiently.

The Situational Judgement Test is often viewed as the easiest section, but it should not be underestimated. One reason is that this is the final section of the examination, and you are likely to be fatigued by this point and therefore more likely to make mistakes. In addition, it is a busy section with a large quantity of scenarios in a short period of time. Finally, it may be that each of the possible answers seem plausible, so it is difficult to identify which one is correct.

In the first set of questions, you have to determine the 'appropriateness' of the options in the given scenario. You will be given the following four options to give as your response.

1. **A very appropriate thing to do:** you should give this answer if it addresses at least one aspect of the scenario; it does not have to be all aspects.
2. **Appropriate, but not ideal:** you should give this answer if it was not an ideal solution, though it could be done, despite not being best practice.
3. **Inappropriate, but not awful:** you should give this answer if it should not be done, though it would not be considered terrible.
4. **A very inappropriate thing to do:** you should give this answer if you should definitely not do this.

In giving a response (i.e. 1–4), always remember that it might not be the only course of action and you should not consider it as such.

In the second set, you need to rate the 'importance' of a number of choices regarding a given scenario. You will be given the following four options to give as your response.

1. **Very important:** you would give this answer if this is vital to take into account.
2. **Important:** you would give this answer if it was important but not vital to take into account.
3. **Of minor importance:** you would give this answer if you should take it into account but it would not matter if it was not considered.
4. **Not important at all:** you would give this answer if you should definitely not be taking this information into account.

When approaching these questions, you should consider:

- the appropriateness or importance of the action
- whether the action actually addresses the problem at hand
- whether there are any possible unintended consequences associated with the action.

In addition to the above, the Situational Judgement section has recently introduced a number of scenarios that are answered through a 'drag-and-drop' format: each question has multiple components and you must drag the correct answer and drop it into each component.

Preparation

Although the UCAT website tries to discourage students from doing any preparation for the test other than sitting the practice tests available online, students who have sat the test in the past have found that the more practice they had on timed IQ-type tests, the better prepared they felt. In this chapter you will find practice questions for each section.

General hints

- Use the practice questions provided on the following pages to familiarise yourself with the type of questions that are asked and the time constraints in the test. It is important to practise the different types of question available so that you can improve your approach to each question type.
- Most candidates have great difficulty completing the sections of the test in the allocated time, so don't panic if you find that this is the case when you are practising questions. The UCAT website provides practice tests that can be completed online, and these give a realistic representation of the level of questioning you will get in the official exam, as well as the timing and the practical aspects of completing tests on a computer.
- There is a point for each right answer, but no points are deducted for wrong answers.

- Try not to leave blanks. If you really can't work out the answer, it is better to eliminate the answers that you know to be wrong and then make your best guess from those that are left. The answers are multiple-choice and, as the test is not negatively marked, it is better to have a go!
- Throughout the test, there is an option to 'flag' questions. If you are struggling with a question, it is best to have a guess at an answer, flag the question and move on. Then, providing you have time remaining at the end, you can easily identify which questions to return to so that you can work through the question again and amend your answer if necessary. This approach will allow you to secure a reasonable number of marks per section on questions that you are confident with (such as those that are shorter and easier to interpret) before spending time on more complicated questions.
- Be aware that you must read the whole screen of the question that you are on, otherwise you cannot move on to the next question or go back to any of the questions you have answered. There are both vertical and horizontal scroll bars.
- Before you start the test, you should be provided with a mini whiteboard, or as is the case in many test centres, a laminated piece of paper. Since the questions must be completed on a computer, there is no option to highlight or underline key points. In this case, the whiteboard or laminated paper provides a useful tool for jotting down any key points or components of calculations. Do not start the test without one, and if you feel it is necessary, ask for more! With the time pressures of the UCAT, even saving time by not having to rub away answers to previous questions can be incredibly valuable.
- It is worth keeping in mind that the precise scoring method is unknown as it is not information that the UCAT consortium shares. However, it is known that the score you obtain roughly corresponds to the number of questions you answer correctly. A maximum score of 900 is incredibly difficult to obtain, yet it is possible to score 900 and make some mistakes. A competitive score is generally viewed as anything above 700, as this is a difficult score to achieve and exceed.
- Finally, it is most important that you stay calm in the test. Prepare yourself, pace yourself and move on if you're struggling with particular questions. It is inevitable that you will find some questions and some sections easier than others. In the same vein, perspective is important – the UCAT score is one aspect of a series of factors that will enable you to study denntistry and is not the single most important part of your application.

Sample questions from each sub-test follow, courtesy of Kaplan Test Prep.

UCAT Verbal Reasoning Practice Questions

Subtest length: 44 questions (11 sets of 4 questions)
Subtest timing: 21 minutes (2 minutes per set)
Sample length: 4 questions
Sample timing: 2 minutes

In 1584, the rediscovery of the works of Tacitus led to the discovery of an old British heroic warrior, Boudicca. No mention is made of Boudicca, also known as Boadicea, in accounts of British history before the Renaissance, but she is referenced in three Roman works: Agricola and The Annals by Tacitus and The Rebellion of Boudicca by Dio. Thus, since the time of Elizabeth I, another of England's great warrior queens, Boudicca has become a part of England's national history.

Boudicca was the wife of Prasutagus, the head of the Iceni tribe in East England. In the year 43 CE when the Romans invaded England, Prasutagus was one of only two Celtic kings to retain some of his power, and the Romans gave him a grant. The Romans later redefined the grant as a loan, and, when Prasutagus died in 60 CE, he left half of his kingdom to Nero in payment, and the remainder to his daughters. When the Romans came to collect, they seized control of the kingdom, and attacked both Boudicca and her daughters.

Boudicca retaliated by attacking the Roman military's British operational base in Camulodunum, while most of the Roman army was away fighting in Wales. boudicca's army drove out the Romans and burned Camulodunum to the ground. Boudicca and her army then attacked Londinium; Boudicca had the city burned to the ground and its entire population massacred. The ancient cities of Camulodunum and Londinium were later rebuilt and have since developed into Colchester and London, respectively.

Today, a bronze statue of Boudicca, commissioned during Victoria's reign and unveiled in 1905, stands alongside Westminster Bridge and the Houses of Parliament. The statue carries an inscription from William Cowper's 1782 poem Boadicea, an Ode: 'Regions Caesar never knew / Thy posterity shall sway.' Ironically, England's early anti-imperialist warrior became a primary cultural symbol for the British Empire, and today she stands over the city she once completely destroyed.

1. The British Empire expanded during Victoria's reign.

A True
B False
C Can't tell

2. Following the Roman invasion, Boudicca's husband was allowed to keep some authority over his kingdom.

A True
B False
C Can't tell

3. Roman forces in ancient Britain were headquartered in what is present-day London.

A True
B False
C Can't tell

4. Some Roman historians took note of a foreign warrior queen.

A True
B False
C Can't tell

UCAT Decision Making Practice Questions

Subtest length: 29 questions (individual items, rather than sets)
Subtest timing: 31 minutes (1 minute per question)
Sample length: 3 questions
Sample timing: 3 minutes

1. *Vaccine K can prevent 88% of cases of Condition I, but cannot prevent 17% of cases of Condition II.*

Vaccine L cannot prevent 11% of cases of Condition I.

Vaccine L can prevent 86% of cases of Condition II.

Based on the success rates **only**, is Vaccine K more effective than Vaccine L at preventing the conditions?

A Yes, because Vaccine K prevents more cases of both conditions.
B Yes, because Vaccine K prevents more cases of Condition I than Vaccine L does.
C No, because Vaccine L is more successful at preventing both conditions.
D No, because Vaccine L is significantly more successful at preventing Condition II, but not Condition I.

2. Should train stations be allowed to charge for the use of the station toilets, which are an essential resource to all passengers who have already paid for a ticket?

Select the strongest argument from the statements below.

A Yes, because the cost of cleaning and maintaining the toilets is considerable.
B Yes, because most toilets are located in a part of the station that can be accessed by anyone, whether or not they have bought a ticket.
C No, because passengers can use the toilets available on the trains.
D No, because not everyone uses the toilets in train stations.

3. Some freshwater fish in the minnow family (Cyprinidae), such as the zebrafish, can regenerate their fins, heart or spinal cord following injury or amputation without any mutation or scarring thanks to fibroblast, a specialised protein that acts as a growth factor.

Place 'Yes' if the conclusion does follow. Place 'No' if the conclusion does not follow.

Minnows can regenerate after an injury without any scars.	
If a fish is a freshwater fish, it contains fibroblast.	
Some members of the family Cyprinidae are freshwater fish.	
Zebrafish can survive any injury by regenerating.	
A protein could allow certain minnows to replace an amputated fin	

UCAT Quantitative Reasoning Practice Questions

Subtest length: 36 questions (9 sets of 4 questions)
Subtest timing: 24 minutes (2 minutes per set)
Sample length: 4 questions
Sample timing: 2 minutes

The table indicates the total cost of renting different types of helicopter for a particular number of hours. Total cost equals the deposit plus the cost of renting per hour. Some information in the table is missing.

Type	Hours	Deposit	Hourly Rate	Total Cost
A	3	—	£500	£1,680
B	5	£240	£650	—
C	8	—	£4,895	£7,600
D	12	£5,675	£1,100	£13,875

1. Ian's total cost of renting a Type B helicopter was £4,790. For how many hours did he rent the helicopter?

A 2
B 3
C 5
D 7
E 9

2. What is the ratio of the total cost of renting a Type A helicopter for 8 hours to the total cost of renting a Type C helicopter for 8 hours?

A 10:19
B 11:20
C 3:5
D 12:19
E 8:11

3. The total cost of a Type D helicopter is discounted by a certain rate if rented for 24 hours. Jenni rents a Type D helicopter for 24 hours, with a total cost of £22,743. How much is the discount?

A 16%
B 18%
C 20%
D 22%
E 24%

4. Type E helicopters have the same deposit as Type A helicopters. The cost per hour of a Type E helicopter is 25% more than for a Type A helicopter. What is the total cost of renting a Type E helicopter for 6 hours?

A £2,430
B £2,520
C £3,930
D £4,080
E £4,200

UCAT Abstract Reasoning Practice Questions

Subtest length: 55 questions (11 sets of 5 questions)
Subtest timing: 13 minutes (1 minute per set)
Sample length: 5 questions
Sample timing: 1 minute

<table>
<tr><th>Set A</th><th>Set B</th></tr>
<tr><td></td><td></td></tr>
</table>

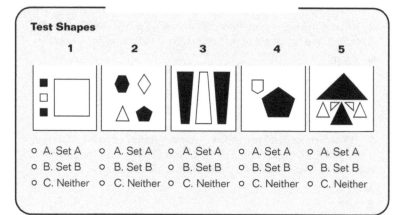

Test Shapes

| 1 | 2 | 3 | 4 | 5 |

○ A. Set A   ○ A. Set A   ○ A. Set A   ○ A. Set A   ○ A. Set A

○ B. Set B   ○ B. Set B   ○ B. Set B   ○ B. Set B   ○ B. Set B

○ C. Neither   ○ C. Neither   ○ C. Neither   ○ C. Neither   ○ C. Neither

UCAT Situational Judgement Practice Questions

Subtest length: 20 scenarios, 2 to 5 questions each (69 questions total)

Subtest timing: 26 minutes (20–30 seconds per scenario, then 10–15 seconds per question)

Sample length: 4 questions

Sample timing: 1 minute

A medical student, Emmet, is completing a patient history as part of his placement at a GP surgery. The patient has previously been treated for emphysema and has difficulty breathing, but he has continued to smoke. The patient mentions that the doctor 'keeps telling me to quit' but insists that he enjoys cigarettes, they help him to relax, and 'you're not taking away my one pleasure in life.' Emmet has experience as a volunteer on a stop smoking campaign, so he feels qualified to engage with the patient on this issue.

How **appropriate** are each of the following responses by Emmet in this situation?

1. Discuss other relaxing activities, such as reading, music or sport, that the patient might enjoy.

A A very appropriate thing to do

B Appropriate, but not ideal

C Inappropriate, but not awful

D A very inappropriate thing to do

2. Tell the patient that he risks shortening his life, with reduced quality of life, if he keeps smoking.

A A very appropriate thing to do

B Appropriate, but not ideal

C Inappropriate, but not awful

D A very inappropriate thing to do

3. Remind the patient that the doctors know best and he would do well to follow their advice.

A A very appropriate thing to do

B Appropriate, but not ideal

C Inappropriate, but not awful

D A very inappropriate thing to do

Verbal Reasoning Practice Questions - Answers

1. C
2. A
3. B
4. A

Decision Making Practice Questions - Answers

1. C
2. B
3. NO; NO; YES; NO; YES

Quantitative Reasoning Practice Questions - Answers

1. D
2. B
3. A
4. C

Abstract Reasoning Practice Questions - Answers

1. A
2. C
3. C
4. A
5. B

Situational Judgement Practice Questions - Answers

1. A
2. B
3. D

All practice questions provided by Kaplan Test Prep, a leading provider of preparation for the UCAT and BMAT.
See www.kaptest.com/ucat to learn more about preparing with Kaplan Test Prep.

UCAT fees

- Test taken in the UK/EU: £75.
- Test taken outside the EU: £120.

This information is accurate at the time of writing, but will be updated in April 2021 for 2022 applications.

BMAT

The BioMedical Admissions Test (BMAT) is an alternative admissions test that is used for a relatively small number of dental, medical and biomedical science courses at selected universities. Currently, only the University of Leeds requires students that apply for dentistry to sit the test. The test, which takes place in November (usually in your school), consists of three sections. In previous years, it has also been possible to sit the test in September (for a higher fee), though due to the pandemic, the September series was cancelled in 2020. It is yet to be determined whether this test will be reinstated for 2021.

If you are taking the BMAT, your school or college will need to register you for the test by 6pm (UK time) on 12 August for the September sitting or 6pm (UK time) on 15 October for the November sitting.

The test can only be taken once per cycle, and many students opt to take the BMAT at the later November date to allow for more preparation time. However, if you have the opportunity to sit the BMAT in September, you will be able to make more informed decisions about your university choices, since you will have the score prior to the UCAS deadline.

In previous years, the BMAT has been a pen and paper exam. However, due to Covid-19, the November sitting was sat using a computer for all candidates except those in Thailand or Singapore. The test format remained the same otherwise. It is yet to be established whether this new testing format will remain in place for 2021.

The BMAT is a very different prospect to the UCAT; it is conducted at your school or college like any GCSE or A-level exam. The test consists of three sections and lasts for two hours in total. Students are advised that it tests both skills and knowledge and as a consequence does require some study. As with the UCAT, it is worth spending as much time as you can preparing for it so that you know exactly what to expect. The BMAT website (www.admissionstesting.org/for-test-takers/bmat/bmat-november or www.admissionstesting.org/for-test-takers/bmat/bmat-september) provides comprehensive information about the structure of the test, guidance on preparing for the test, as well as details of the scientific content that will be tested. There is also a number of practice papers included that will help you to get used to the question style and format as well as the timing of each of the sections. There are also numerous other websites and preparation course providers that provide useful practice materials and support.

The three sections of the test are as follows:

1. thinking skills
2. scientific knowledge and applications
3. writing task.

The structure and layout of each section is described below.

1. Thinking skills

The Thinking Skills section lasts for one hour and consists of 32 multiple-choice questions. The test is designed to demonstrate your ability to solve problems and understand arguments. This part of the test is very similar in style to UCAT and uses the same sorts of skills as the verbal, quantitative and abstract reasoning sections.

For the 2020 exams, the Thinking Skills section was updated so that it did not include questions that test data analysis and inference. In previous years, students had to complete questions that assessed whether they could understand verbal, statistical and graphical information. It is assumed that this update will remain in place for 2021.

BMAT® Thinking Skills Practice Questions

DIRECTIONS (for full test):

Answer every question. Points are awarded for correct answers only. There are no penalties for incorrect answers.

All questions are worth 1 mark.

3. The media frequently shares stories about the supposed dangers of screen time for children and teenagers, but there has been little discussion of the appropriate amount of screen time for adults. Recent research indicates that adults average 11 hours of screen time per day, which means that adults spend most of our waking time looking at screens. That figure has increased from nine and a half hours four years ago. Of the current figures, 43% of daily screen time is spent watching TV, 21% using smartphones, and 7% using tablets. This data underlines the fact that concerns about people spending too much time looking at smartphones are misguided, since adults actually spend significantly more time watching TV.

Which of the following is the best statement of the conclusion in the argument above?

A No one can say how much daily screen time is suitable for adults.

B It is unwarranted to worry that someone's smartphone screen time is excessive.

C Compared to smartphone usage, watching TV takes up more of the average adult's day.

D Adults spend more and more time looking at screens each year.

E There is not enough awareness of the dangers of screen time for adults.

4. The clocks in Beematia use an unusual format to indicate the time. Beematia uses a 24-hour clock in the format mm:hh, in which mm indicates the number of minutes to the next hour (hh). For example, 12:05 indicates the time is 12 minutes before 5am. Each day in Beematia has 24 hours and each hour has 60 minutes.

Srinand is visiting Beematia, and the clocks in his hotel room indicate the time in this format.

The clock in the hotel room says 19:22 when Srinand goes to sleep. When he wakes up, the clock reads 22:07.

For how long has Srinand slept?

A 2 hours, 45 minutes

B 7 hours, 41 minutes

C 8 hours, 57 minutes

D 9 hours, 3 minutes

E 10 hours, 19 minutes

2. Scientific Knowledge and Applications

The Scientific Knowledge section lasts for 30 minutes and consists of 27 multiple-choice questions. This section tests your ability to apply GCSE-standard scientific knowledge and, as such, requires a knowledge of biology, chemistry, physics and mathematics. This marks a departure from the skills required for UCAT and is the only section that requires revision of scientific content. The BMAT website provides a specification and an electronic 'revision' guide to allow candidates to prepare the basics needed for this section (www.admissionstestingservice.org/for-test-takers/bmat/preparing-for-bmat/section-2-preparation).

BMAT® Scientific Knowledge and Applications Practice Questions

DIRECTIONS (for full test):

Answer every question. Points are awarded for correct answers only. There are no penalties for incorrect answers. All questions are worth 1 mark. Some questions have more than 1 correct answer. Read carefully to ensure that you select the appropriate number of answers. Calculators are not permitted during any portion of the test.

1. Freckles are autosomal dominant, meaning that a child with at least one dominant allele will have freckles. Children with a recessive genotype will not have freckles.

A husband and wife both have freckles, but their first child does not have freckles.

What is the probability that their next child will have freckles?

A 0%

B 12.5%

C 25%

D 37.5%

E 50%

F 62.5%

G 75%

H 100%

3. The first five hexagonal numbers are 1, 6, 15, 28 and 45.

The difference between the first and second hexagonal numbers is 5.

The difference between the second and third hexagonal numbers is 9.

The difference between the third and fourth hexagonal numbers is 13.

The difference between the fourth and fifth hexagonal numbers is 17.

All the hexagonal numbers follow this pattern.

The difference between the rth hexagonal number and the $(r + 3)$th hexagonal number is 363.

What is the value of r?

A 28

B 29

C 30

D 31

E 32

3. Writing Task

The final stage is the Writing Task, which lasts for 30 minutes and requires you to choose one task from a possible three questions. This is predominantly designed to see how you can arrange your ideas and then communicate them in written form. There are strict limits on the amount of space available, so one of the main purposes of this section is to test your ability to write clearly and concisely and get your points across without waffling.

BMAT® Writing Practice Questions

Time: 30 MINUTES

DIRECTIONS (for full test):

Answer only one task from the choice of four essay titles. You must write your answer by hand, and are limited to a space consisting of one side of A4. You are permitted to make any preparatory notes as needed, but time spent on such notes counts against the 30 minutes allowed for the essay. In this task, you are expected to show how well you can order and explore ideas, and convey these ideas in clear, effective writing. You may not use dictionaries or any other reference books or resources. Essays are assigned a numerical score. To achieve a top mark, you must address all aspects of the question and write compellingly with few errors in logic or in use of English.

1. **All 16-year-olds should be required to complete first aid training, as part of the National Curriculum.**

Write an essay in which you address the following points:

What are the advantages in training all 16-year-olds in how to give CPR and deal with heart attacks, strokes and other major injuries? What are the drawbacks of requiring such training? To what extent do you agree that some first aid training should be compulsory, and at what age?

2. **Research is what I'm doing when I don't know what I'm doing.** (Wernher von Braun, German scientist, 1912–1977)

Write an essay in which you address the following points:

Explain what this statement means. Argue that a scientist can only undertake research with a clear goal or objective in mind. To what extent do you agree with von Braun that research is possible, or preferable, when scientists don't know what they're doing?

BMAT® Thinking Skills Practice Answers

3. B

4. C

BMAT® Scientific Knowledge and Applications Practice Answers

1. G

3. B

All practice questions provided by Kaplan Test Prep, a leading provider of preparation for the UCAT and BMAT. See www.kaptest.com/bmat to learn more about preparing with Kaplan Test Prep.

Tips for BMAT

- Familiarity with the basic structure of the test is good preparation, so make sure that you utilise the past paper questions available on the website. This is especially useful for Section 1, which requires the development of skills for the aptitude test.
- You can revise for Section 2 of the test as it covers biology, chemistry, physics and maths to GCSE standard.
- As with the UCAT, the majority of candidates do not complete all sections in the test so don't worry if you don't. Ensure that you have tried the practice tests first so that you understand the timing of the test. Try to answer as many questions as you can but do not worry if you do not get to the end of each section. If you are short on time, make sure that you do not leave an answer blank – the test is not negatively marked, so it is worth having a go!
- Practise writing the essays under timed conditions and using BMAT test paper, since there is a space constraint. Where possible, get advice from a teacher about how best to structure your essays and make best use of the time and space available.
- You can access a specification for the BMAT exam, so it is advisable that you review this carefully as part of your preparation.
- In Sections 1 and 2, there is a point for each right answer, but no points are deducted for wrong answers.
- In Section 3, each of the essays is double marked and there is a mark for the quality of written English presentation.
- It might be obvious, but the best thing you can do is stay calm. If you have put in the time to practise beforehand, then you have prepared as best you can. Do not ruin your chances by letting nerves get in your way.

Dates

A list of important dates regarding the BMAT exam can be found at www.bmat.org.uk. For 2021 entry in 2021 (based on 2019/20 entry timescale), the most important ones are as follows:

- registration opens: 1 September
- registration deadline: 1 October
- late registration deadline: 15 October
- takes place on: 4 November
- results released: 27 November.

NB: These dates are subject to change and the BMAT website should be checked in the run up to the registration dates.

Deferred entry

Some admissions tutors may be happy to consider students who take a gap year; however, if you are considering following this route, you first need to make sure that you contact your prospective universities in order to see if they would be willing to accept a deferral. If you receive positive feedback about this route, the next step is to ensure that you have plans in place to use the time constructively. A year spent watching daytime TV is not going to impress anybody, whereas independent travelling, charity or voluntary work either at home or abroad, work experience or a responsible job will all indicate that you have used the time to develop independence and maturity.

Having a job during your gap year in somewhere like a shop or a bar may seem like a good idea and is certainly better than sitting around doing nothing all the time; however, if you wish to demonstrate your ongoing commitment to pursuing dentistry as a career, then you should concentrate on getting further experience in a job or placement directly related to the field.

You can either apply for deferred entry when you submit your UCAS application, in which case you need to outline your plans clearly in your personal statement, or apply in September following the publication of your A level results. If you expect to be predicted the right grades, and the feedback from your school or college is that you will be given a good reference, you should apply for deferred entry. On the other hand, if you are advised by your referee that you are unlikely to be considered, you should give yourself more time to work with your referees by waiting until you have your A level results.

Dental timeline

Figure 1 (opposite) shows what you will need to be aware of over the course of your A level studies and gives an overview of the timings of some of the various tasks that you should plan for if you are to maximise your chances of gaining entry into a dental school.

As you can see, your main task in year 12 is to start researching your courses and options, organising and carrying out work experience and then preparing your personal statement. The summer between year 12 and year 13 should be used to continue building your work experience as well as registering and preparing for the UCAT.

In year 13 you must hit the ground running, because the UCAT and your UCAS application must be finished by early October. At the same time, you must also ensure that you stay on top of your studies so you maximise your chances of achieving the A grades you will need, and you should also start preparing for interview and practising your interview skills.

Once your final exams are finished at the end of the year, it is simply a matter of waiting for your results so you can see whether you have secured a place.

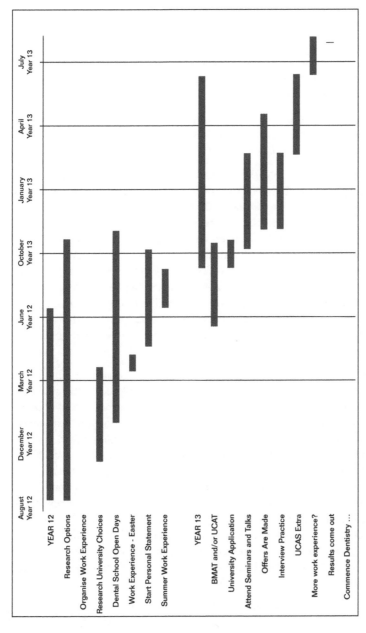

Figure 1 Timeline to guide your application to study dentistry

5 | Personal statement

In spite of the fluctuations in application numbers for dentistry in recent years, the demand is still extremely high when compared to most other undergraduate courses. So, what exactly is the impact of sustained high demand for places?

Firstly, there is a continued requirement for very high A level grades, but, alongside this, there is an increased level of scrutiny of all the other elements of your application.

Your application is likely to be received by the university and considered along with many others at the same time. For example, Manchester Dental School receives around 700 applications each year and has to select around 350 applicants to be called for interview. Of those who apply, there will be some who are automatically rejected as they do not fulfil all the entry criteria; for example, not meeting the GCSE grade requirements. Following this, it is down to the admissions team to try to select whom to interview from the remaining candidates. Many of the applicants who are still being considered at this stage will have excellent GCSE profiles, outstanding predicted A level grades and a strong UCAT (or BMAT, in the case of Leeds) performance. So how do the selectors make their choices?

When it comes to distinguishing between highly qualified candidates, one of the most important factors that is considered is the personal statement. If this is badly worded, littered with errors or lacking detail about the attributes and experiences of the candidate, your application will stand a chance of being rejected without being taken further. Ultimately, this means that the more thought that you give to your UCAS application and personal statement, the better they will be and the greater your chance of being asked to come in for an interview and being made a conditional offer. Remember that the selectors will not know about the things that you have forgotten to say: they can get an impression of you only from what is in the application. We have come across many good students who never secured an interview simply because their personal statement did not adequately reflect their skills and experience.

Note that only a small proportion of applicants will be interviewed, so while it's important to prepare for the interview it's vital that you make your personal statement and overall application as strong as it possibly can be to maximise the chance of you being called to interview in the first place.

The following sections will tell you more about what the selectors are looking for in a personal statement, and how you can avoid common mistakes.

Personal statement basics

When constructing your personal statement, there are several important things that you need to consider. First, your personal statement needs to be no more than 47 lines or 4,000 characters, including spaces; this is a strict limit and so you need to ensure that you are as close to this as possible. You must then consider the key themes of your personal statement, which are:

- why you want to be a dentist
- what you have done to gain work experience and voluntary work placements
- what experiences have particularly stood out to you and why
- what your academic interests are and how these have furthered your desire to pursue dentistry
- what you have done to develop the skills needed to become a dentist
- what you have done outside of academic studies to develop your skills.

The personal statement is your opportunity to demonstrate to the selectors that you are fully committed to studying dentistry and have the right motivation and personal qualities to do so successfully. A typical personal statement takes time and effort to get right: don't expect perfection after one draft. At each stage of the process, take time to read through your statement, and ask yourself the question: 'Does it sound like me?' If not, redraft it. You should also take the time to get your academic advisers or teachers to give you feedback at each stage; this will ensure you stay on the right track.

Sections of the personal statement

Why dentistry?

This should be your first section and will outline to the admissions tutors your motivation for wanting to study dentistry. A high proportion of UCAS applications contain stock phrases such as: 'From an early age I have wanted to be a dentist because it is the only career that combines my love of science with the chance to work with people.' Not only do admissions tutors get bored with reading such statements, remarks like these are also clearly untrue: if you think about it, there are many careers that combine science and working with people, including medicine, teaching, pharmacy, physiotherapy and nursing. Nevertheless, the basic idea of this sentence may well apply to you. If so, you need to personalise it. You could mention an incident that first got you interested in dentistry – a visit to your own dentist, a conversation with a family friend, a talk or lesson at school or something you witnessed during your work experience, for instance. You should also ensure that you avoid giving reasons relating to money or status; any mention of wanting to be a dentist so that you can earn £200,000 a year is an almost guaranteed way of being rejected!

It is a common misconception that you need to begin your personal state-ment with an inspirational quotation or grand statement; again, admissions tutors get bored of students trying to squeeze in lines from books, poems or films that have no real meaning to the applicant. What an admissions tutor would rather see is a statement of the genuine reasons why you want to study dentistry, written in clear, uncomplicated English.

Another common pitfall in the first paragraph is taking up valuable space with an explanation about what the subject is about or what the profes-sion entails. For example: 'Dentistry is a highly regarded profession that requires a high degree of manual dexterity and attention to detail.' Remember that the people reading your statement know exactly what the profession is about and so do not need to be lectured on it! Instead, you need to take the time to explain about your own interest in the profession and why you feel compelled to follow this career path.

What work experience and voluntary work have you undertaken?

This section is important to demonstrate that you gained something from your work experience and voluntary placements, and that they have given you an insight into the profession. Start by talking about your dental-specific experiences. You should give an indication of the length of time you spent at each placement and the impressions you gained. You could comment on what aspects of dentistry attract you, on what you found interesting, or on something that you hadn't expected. But remember that this is not a shopping list; you are not simply reeling off experience after experience; you are expected to provide deeper reflec-tion about what you have seen.

Beyond this, you should also mention any other work experience or voluntary work you have had in a caring or clinical role and what you learned from it. Although you may not think of these sorts of experi-ences as being relevant, they can often demonstrate to an admissions tutor good interpersonal skills or commitment and dedication.

Here is a sample description of a student's work experience that would probably not impress the admissions team.

'I spent three days at my local dental practice. I saw some patients having fillings, and a man whose false teeth didn't fit. It was very interesting.'

In contrast, the example below would be much more convincing because it is clear that the student was interested in what was happening.

'During my two weeks at the Smith and Smith Dental Clinic, I shadowed two dentists and a hygienist. I watched a range of treatments including fillings, a root canal, extractions and orthodontic treatment. I found particularly interesting the fact that, although both dentists had very different personalities, they both related well to the patients, who seemed to find them very reassuring. A number of things surprised me; in particular, how demanding a dentist's day is.'

It will be far easier to write this section of your personal statement if you kept notes in a reflective journal during your work experience as discussed in Chapter 2. Look back over what you wrote and use your thoughts and experiences as a stimulus for this section. With luck, the selectors may pick up on these experiences at interview and ask you to expand on some of your comments.

Following this, you should discuss the experiences you have had while undertaking any voluntary work. Any type of voluntary placement is a useful addition to your statement, but ongoing work in a care-based or clinical setting really boosts your profile. Opportunities often exist in care homes, children's hospices and hospitals and it is worth trying to contribute regularly over a long period of time rather than carrying it out for just a week or two. This type of experience can help you get an insight into patient care and the communication side of the profession and gives a really good opportunity to discuss how your interpersonal skills have developed while working with people. As with any dental work experience, you should make a note of any key experiences that you have had and what they have taught you, as this can then be commented on in your personal statement.

In coming years, as students across the country feel the impact of Covid-19 on their work experience and voluntary work, it may be that there will be less to discuss in this section of the personal statement. If you find yourself in the position where you have had no opportunity to develop a work-experience profile due to the pandemic, take the opportunity to discuss anything else that you have done to inform your understanding of the profession. For example, you may have completed one of the many online courses about dentistry that are available on the internet; you may have spoken to a current dentist via an internet communication platform; or you may have carried out other types of voluntary work that are more Covid-secure than working in a care home.

Your academic interests

It is important for your personal statement to contain information about your academic interests and how they have furthered your desire to study dentistry. This may be related to some topics or practical skills that have been of particular interest to you over the course of your A level studies, or to an interesting article you have read in a newspaper or journal, or to something engaging you heard in a lecture. Whatever it is, it will help to demonstrate your desire to pursue the course, as long as you make it relevant to dentistry and put in sufficient detail. In so many personal statements this section struggles to get beyond 'I enjoyed learning about the human body' and 'I enjoy using different apparatus in practical work'; however, this is too generic to be meaningful. Keeping a journal over a long period of time of any wider reading that is relevant to dentistry will help this section to genuinely reflect what your interests are rather than being based on what you have panic read the week before submitting your application.

Evidence of developing skills and personal qualities

The person reading your UCAS application has to decide two things: whether you have the right skills and personal qualities to become a successful dentist, and whether you will be able to cope with and contribute to dental school life. To be a successful dentist, you need (among other things!) to:

- successfully pass your undergraduate studies
- have good interpersonal skills and get on with a wide range of people
- be able to work under pressure and cope with stress
- have well-developed manual skills.

How, then, does the person reading your personal statement know whether you have the qualities they are looking for? What you must remember is that the admissions tutor doesn't know you, so you have to give lots of evidence of how you have demonstrated and developed these qualities. Some of the things they may be looking for are:

- skill development during work experience/voluntary work
- positions of responsibility
- work in the local community
- an ability to get on with people
- participation in activities involving manual dexterity
- participation in team events
- involvement in school plays or concerts.

What they don't want to hear is how you have demonstrated interpersonal skills by going out with your friends every weekend or how you have improved your manual dexterity by playing PlayStation 4 games!

The selectors will be aware that some schools offer more to their students in the way of activities and responsibilities than others. However, even if there are very few opportunities made available to you through your school, you must still find ways to gain experience and develop your skills. You don't have to have been captain of the rugby team or gone on a three-month expedition to Borneo to be considered, but you do need to be able to demonstrate that you have made efforts to participate in a range of worthwhile activities.

Remember, however, that while evidence of all these skills and extra interests is extremely important, it will not compensate for lower grades, so having a strong academic profile and getting high grades still remain the most important aspects of your application.

Weak and strong personal statements

The box below gives an example of a personal statement I have constructed based on experience of reading through what students write. It is made up of a combination of some good ideas, points that need to be expanded on, and things not to say! Overall, as you will probably notice, this would be considered a weak statement and would be unlikely to lead to an offer being made.

DO NOT COPY ANY PARTS OF THESE PERSONAL STATEMENTS!

You should use these examples to give you an idea of structure and the type of content you may want to include, but universities have sophisticated software to detect copied parts of personal statements so do not be tempted! Your personal statement should be personal to you, and, above all else, it should be honest.

Personal statement: Example 1 (character count: 1,859)

The role of a dentist is to look after the oral health of the patient and perform procedures such as root canals and fillings.

I first wanted to study medicine, but after discussing with my friend, I realised that dentistry was a much easier subject and would give me a chance to earn far more money. I have always liked science and so I think that dentistry would suit me perfectly. I really like the idea of giving people a perfect smile as I believe that a smile is a light in the window of the soul.

In my work experience I mainly watched the dentist see patients and observed procedures such as: fillings, root canals, scale and polish, denture fitting, tooth extraction and fitting of crowns and

---

bridges. My voluntary work was really good and showed me how to work with people.

During my A levels, I have enjoyed studying my subjects. In chemistry, I have been really good at practical work and in biology, I really enjoy looking at the human body. I have not really enjoyed studying maths, but I have loved learning about modern European history and the events in the aftermath of the First World War that directly contributed to Hitler coming to power and the Second World War. I have found it fascinating how the political super-powers of the USA and USSR emerged from the aftermath of the war.

I also have a number of interests outside of school. I like relaxing and enjoy watching TV. I also like going out with my mates at the weekend. I play football in a local league, read science fiction books, play the piano, go to the gym and listen to music. I also have a Saturday job which gives me some extra money to spend when I go out with my mates. An exclusive ubiquity of mine is that I am contented with mixing my social with my educational life at length, making the two important factors in my life none the less unabridged.

Personal statement: Example 1 raises a number of interesting points.

1. **It is too short.**
   This statement is just under 1,900 characters. The limit is 4,000 characters (including spaces) and you should aim to use as much of this as possible. Anything significantly below the character count will make a negative impression on the admissions tutors.

2. **It lacks detail and specific examples and has no reflection.**
   The candidate has got the right idea about the structure and attempted the key sections. However, it is very light on actual detail and doesn't really expand on any of the points made or give specific examples. When discussing work experience, go into detail about what you witnessed and reflect on what you learned. When giving details of what you are studying, be specific about topics you have enjoyed. This will give the admissions tutor a much greater insight into who you are and the skills you possess.

3. **It is not very personal.**
   This could be about any number of candidates applying to dentistry. Make sure your personal statement has evidence and experiences to show an admissions tutor who you really are and what you are genuinely interested in.

4. **It has a negative tone in relation to dentistry.**
   Unfortunately, many personal statements contain negative points about things that an applicant hasn't enjoyed studying or things they might not like about the career. These are sometimes included due to

a misguided need to be brutally honest, but this really is not necessary. The overall tone should be optimistic and positive throughout.

5. **It wastes time telling them about dentistry.**
    Statements can often waste time by listing facts about dentistry or what dentists do. Remember that the people reading your statement will know all of this. Use the space instead to illustrate from your own experiences that you possess the qualities and skills that dentists need.

6. **It mentions money and potential earnings.**
    Although most dentistry applicants will have thought about how much money they will be making at some point, it is not something that needs to be highlighted in your personal statement. Your reasons for studying dentistry need to run much deeper than this if you are going to get into dental school.

7. **It seems too focused on cosmetic dentistry.**
    Lots of people fixate on the idea of specialising in cosmetic dentistry. However, dentistry is a far broader discipline and a personal statement should really reflect an understanding of this fact.

8. **It employs overused, repeated stock phrases.**
    Similes such as the smile being a light in the window of the soul are clichéd and can make an admissions tutor question whether your statement is an accurate picture of who you are. If you genuinely want to express an idea like this, think of how you could expand on it in your own words to make it more meaningful.

9. **It vaguely uses the idea of practical work to demonstrate manual dexterity.**
    If you are going to use the example of science practicals to demonstrate your manual dexterity, give specific examples of those you have enjoyed or apparatus you have used. You must also try to think of other activities that have helped you demonstrate these skills outside of your A level curriculum.

10. **It is very itemised.**
    It can be very easy to simply reduce your work experience and extracurricular activities to a long list. Take time to explain what you gained from each of your placements or interests and how they benefit your application. In addition to this, avoid mentioning mundane interests such as going out with friends and watching TV, because they tell the admissions tutor very little about you.

11. **It demonstrates the most passion when discussing an unrelated subject.**
    The only place in this statement that really comes close to the level of detail required is when it discusses A level History. Although it is great that this section uses lots of detail, the space would be better used discussing something more closely related to dentistry.

12. **It swallows a dictionary/thesaurus at the end.**
    Beware of overusing a dictionary or thesaurus. Obviously, you want your English to be as good as possible, but make sure that what you have written makes sense and sounds like you.

Although this statement is poor, it would not need much effort to make it a reasonable attempt, as the basic structure is fine. Your first attempt at writing a personal statement will probably be difficult and might not produce great results; however, it is important that you get feedback on your efforts and then redraft the statement as many times as necessary. The best personal statements can take up to 10 drafts to get completely right! Some suggestions for changes that would be worth making are shown in the following box.

The role of the dentist is to look after the oral health of the patient and perform procedures such as root canals and fillings. [*Develop this. It is a waste of time regurgitating what an admissions tutor will already know about dentistry as a career, so instead talk about why helping patients to look after their oral health interests you.*]

I first wanted to study medicine, but after discussing with my friend, I realised that dentistry was a much easier subject and would give me a chance to earn far more money. [*Do not mention other careers you have thought about. Focus on the one you are applying for.*] I have always liked science and so I think that dentistry would suit me perfectly. [*Expand on this to give much more detail about your reasons for wanting to pursue dentistry.*] I really like the idea of giving people a perfect smile as I believe that a smile is a light in the window of the soul. [*This is a real cliché, so think about what you want to say and put it into your own words to make it clear.*]

In my work experience I mainly watched the dentist see patients and observed procedures such as: fillings, root canals, scale and polish, denture fitting, tooth extraction and fitting of crowns and bridges. [*This lacks any real details about what your observations were and what it made you think about the profession. Make sure that any description is followed by careful reflection. What did you see that was of particular interest to you? What shocked you?*] My voluntary work was really good and showed me how to work with people. [*Give details. What did you do? When did you do it? How long was it for?*]

During my A levels, I have enjoyed studying my subjects. In chemistry, I have been really good at practical work and in biology, I really enjoy looking at the human body. [*Give specific detail. Which areas of biology and chemistry did you enjoy and why? Which practicals did you enjoy carrying out?*] I have not really enjoyed studying maths ... [*Don't put anything negative.*] ... but I have loved learning about modern European history and the events of the First World War that directly contributed to Hitler coming to power and the Second World War. In particular, I have found it

---

fascinating how the political superpowers of the USA and USSR emerged from the aftermath of the war. [*This detail is great, but the characters need to be used to expand on areas that are more directly related to dentistry.*]

I also have a number of interests outside of school. I like relaxing and enjoy watching TV. I also like going out with my mates at the weekend. I play football in a local league, read science fiction books, play the piano, go to the gym and listen to music. I also have a Saturday job which gives me some extra money to spend when I go out with my mates. [*Ordinary interests are fine, but don't spend too much time discussing them. If you do want to put these things in, try to link to key skills that you have developed by doing them.*] An exclusive ubiquity of mine is that I am contented with mixing my social with my educational life at length making the two important factors in my life none the less unabridged. [*This is a typical thesaurus overload sentence that makes no sense. This can also come about from copying from other personal statements on the internet.*]

Here are two examples of much better personal statements based on those written by two students who both secured entry onto dental courses. Each demonstrates clarity and focus, and what comes through is the enthusiasm that the candidates have for dentistry.

Personal statement: Example 2 (character count: 3,977)

Being very close to my family, my passion for dentistry grew from an experience involving them. My younger sister had many self-esteem issues, many of which stemmed from her teeth. She underwent a course of orthodontic treatment, and now she has an enviably perfect smile. My sister's transformation was simply astonishing to me, and I realise it was not merely limited to her appearance. While I attended my dentist regularly, I had not paid much thought to the extent of their abilities. However, this miraculous change in a physical state that had existed since birth was a turning point for me. Recalling sitting in the visitor's chair, observing the close relationship established between my sister and the orthodontist, their reassurance and accurate diagnosis, and how the dental practice focused its efforts purely on providing patient satisfaction, was where the true purpose of it all became apparent. Improving the life of another became the predominant factor in my decision of this career. Dentistry is ever-expanding, something I witnessed at the Dental Show at the NEC

Birmingham. This highlighted the opportunity for further specialisation, thus providing an emotionally and physically engaging career through improving the wellbeing of others.

The human body's biological intricacies are truly captivating. I investigated them deeper by completing an EPQ, discussing the problem and history of Odontophobia. This was aided by completing an online course provided by the University of Sussex. Alongside this, studying religious studies at GCSE level and discussing topics such as euthanasia, I can maintain an argued moral position while empathising with those belonging to others.

Undertaking work experience over four weeks intensified my passion for dentistry. I shadowed a dentist in a high-volume practice based in a socially deprived area. This granted a unique perspective, where factors I had not previously considered were highly important. I observed the job's demands and the role of a dentist in providing high-quality care. Further, I learnt the importance of the role of individuals within a dental practice, such as the practice manager, who is responsible for such tasks as the correct disposal of hazardous waste and ensuring that the nurses are trained correctly. Taking this into my volunteering role in a charity shop, my communication skills have improved as I am now more structured in my responses to customers. Having to sort through donations and quickly determine whether they are suitable for sale and price them has improved my decision making. I also regularly assist my sibling in her cupcake business, decorating intricate cupcakes, thus maintaining high manual dexterity skills, which are vital in dentistry.

Despite my various commitments, I still aim to find time to engage in leisurely activities. Throughout my childhood, and to this day, I have shown an interest in sport, particularly football. Recently, I was offered a trial with Sandwell Academy at county level, but believed that my time could be better utilised volunteering and continuing to play football at a slightly lower level. Competing in a football tournament that took place in Germany, we narrowly missed out on success. While we were there, I had the opportunity to lead a training session with a group of younger children who could not speak English; but with the aid of the universal language of football, we undertook a rigorous training session, which they thoroughly enjoyed. I also enjoy creative writing, shown by one of my short stories reaching the long-list of a Radio 2 writing competition.

I firmly believe that I would be suited to dentistry, not just as a degree but as a career. Dentistry is a labour in which tough challenges are inevitable. Nevertheless, I thoroughly welcome them as opportunities to test myself and advance as both a professional and as a person.

Personal statement: Example 3 (character count: 3,993)

The effect a dentist can have on a teenager's wellbeing is profound. I experienced this first-hand when undergoing orthodontic treatment at age 16. My outlook changed over 18 months, from being self-conscious to an outgoing individual. At this point, I became aware of how fulfilling the work of a dentist can be, and it initiated my interest to consider it as a future career. Just as importantly, it prompted me to take up work experience, where my intentions to study dentistry were confirmed.

Over the two weeks I spent in a local NHS dental practice, I was able to follow many patients from the first consultation to the completion of treatment. It was rewarding to watch as each problem was rectified systematically, as with the methodical steps of a root canal treatment. An area that I found fascinating was the importance of preventative healthcare – for instance, the idea that thumb sucking in children can cause malocclusion, and simple, proactive steps such as education for parents could prevent this. This year, I have decided to read further into this and to complete an EPQ titled: 'To what extent do habits in young children lead to the need for orthodontic treatment.'

I witnessed professionalism in the holistic approach of the dentist, and I recognised the importance of composure for a dentist. During a difficult extraction, I watched a carious tooth break, leading to each root needing to be drilled apart and extracted separately with Cryer's elevators. I observed how the dentist maintained trust and patient satisfaction by allaying the patient's initial panic, who was visibly put at ease. I also shadowed dentists and maxillofacial surgeons in theatre, spent time with orthodontic specialists, and learnt to cast study models in a dental laboratory.

For over a year I volunteered as a Health Care Support Worker at the Douglas Macmillan Hospice, where my role was to provide personal care for terminally ill patients; this was daunting at first, however I took the opportunity to empathise with patients. Interacting with people of different ages and abilities, I have gained invaluable communication skills, for example, patience and clarity of speech.

As part of National Citizen Service, I had the opportunity to work with people recently granted refugee status. Teaching English and helping to mentor, I was challenged with many language barriers; but with the help of body language and hand gestures, I was able to overcome these. Completing my DofE Gold as team leader, I built a good rapport with my colleagues: having an open mind to suggestions while always respecting others' opinions. As a school prefect, I have exercised self-discipline and responsibility, with a willingness to help others. I have achieved merit in Grade 8 piano, which has required a great deal of concentration and commitment.

My years of training in swimming, resulting in selection to the Midlands Regional squad, have helped me to focus on my progress and determination to do well. Furthermore, I have demonstrated my capacity for leadership and teamwork as a county-level rugby player. Team and individual sport have given me physical and mental stability and fostered a strong work ethic. I have also worked in a bicycle shop, where I helped to repair and assemble mountain bikes while gaining an insight into the running of a business. The manual dexterity involved when using tools and small parts was aided by my existing manual skills developed on the piano. This culminated in the ability to build my own mountain bike – which has yet to fall apart!

Upon receiving my A levels results I was disappointed, but I have proven to myself that I have what it takes to succeed in previous challenges. I understand that a career in dentistry involves a lifelong path of learning and development, which I know is not easy. However, I believe that my drive to succeed, the experiences I have gained and my ability to strive to better myself, will make me a successful dental student.

Final points to remember before submitting your personal statement

- Your personal statement will require careful proofreading to ensure that your spelling, punctuation and grammar are sound and that there are no careless errors that have crept in. Beware of solely relying on computer software or internet-based applications to do the checking for you; they will often misinterpret some of your phrases and perpetuate errors.
- It is worth getting another person to check your statement before submission. If you have been through it many times, it is unlikely you will spot errors that might be glaringly obvious to somebody else. However, beware of getting too many people to work on it as you can often end up with so many opinions that it can be hard to incorporate all of the ideas.
- Keep a copy of your statement so that you can use it as a reminder of what you have written. Remember that it is possible that an interviewer could use your personal statement as a starting point for a question, so you must be aware of what you said.
- Make sure that you are able to talk about all of the individual elements of your application at interview if needed. If there is anything you have included that you would not be able to discuss, remove it before submission.

University of Bristol

'Given the very large number of applications we receive each year from applicants who have achieved or are predicted to achieve high grades, we necessarily place substantial emphasis upon the quality of the personal statement. We look for:

- Evidence of work experience and motivation and understanding of dentistry
- Evidence of teamwork or non-academic achievement
- Evidence of contribution to society.'

Source: www.bristol.ac.uk/study/media/undergraduate/admissions-statements/2020/dentistry.pdf
Reprinted with kind permission of the University of Bristol

Queen's University Belfast

Personal statements are not scored as part of the selection process and the following general factors are taken into account when considering applications:
(i) Candidates are expected to state explicitly that Dentistry is their career choice. (Please note that an applicant cannot normally be considered for both Medicine and Dentistry.)
(ii) There should be evidence of commitment and motivation to follow a career in Dentistry.
(iii) Work experience in a dental clinical setting is not a requirement for admission, however, applicants should state what they have done to find out about a career in Dentistry.

Application checklist

- Do you have at least two weeks' dental-based work experience?
- If Covid-19 has impacted your ability to secure work experience, have you undertaken other activities to develop your knowledge and understanding of dentistry?
- Do you have evidence of ongoing voluntary work?
- Do you meet the GCSE entrance requirements for your chosen universities?
- Are you studying the correct combination of A level subjects?
- Are you on target for at least AAA?
- Have you researched the different dental schools and their courses?
- Have you been to university open days (virtual or in person)?
- Have you registered for/completed the UCAT and/or BMAT?
- Does your personal statement demonstrate the commitment, skills and attributes that the university is looking for?

What happens next?

- Immediately after UCAS receives your application, you will receive an email confirming receipt of your application. It is vital that you check this information carefully and inform UCAS if there are any inaccuracies. A common mistake is to select the foundation year – the 'pre-dental' year – rather than the start of the course proper, so make sure you haven't done this. Remember, you will be able to access your application at all times through the UCAS Track system using the same personal ID, username and password that you used to apply.
- As soon as UCAS processes your application, your prospective universities can access it, but they will be unable to see the other courses and universities that you have applied to, as long as they are not at the same institution. Once a university has accessed your application, it may contact you to acknowledge your application; however, not all universities bother doing this, so don't worry if you don't hear from them initially.
- The next stage is to wait to hear from the universities you applied to. If the universities feel that you have met their criteria, you will be invited to attend an interview. Some dental schools interview on a first-come, first-served basis, while others wait until all applications are in before deciding whom to interview. It is not uncommon for students to hear nothing until after Christmas, so don't panic if you aren't contacted straight away.
- If your application is unsuccessful, you will receive a notification from UCAS telling you that you have been rejected by one or more of the dental schools. If this happens, don't despair: you may hear better news from another of the schools that you applied to. If you ultimately end up with four rejections, you should take the opportunity to carefully reassess whether dentistry is a realistic career ambition for you and whether there were any parts of your application that let you down. If you still feel that dentistry is for you, take the opportunity to strengthen any aspects of your application that were weak, for example undertaking further work experience. Under no circumstances should you give up and decide that it is no longer worth working hard in your academic studies; this will only reduce your chances of making a successful application the following year.
- Note that going through Clearing is not an option that you should bank on for entry into dentistry. Places are limited and often over-subscribed, and more offers are made than there are places. There can be the odd exception on a year-to-year basis where a few places are available through Clearing (although these are not usually advertised on Clearing lists); however, under no circumstances should you rely on any such places becoming available.

6 | What makes a successful interview?

Once you've submitted your UCAS application, you must wait to hear from each of the universities you have applied to. If you meet their entry criteria and they feel that your application is strong in the areas they deem to be most important, they may call you for interview. The universities use interviews to find out firsthand whether the picture painted by your application is accurate and to investigate whether you have the skills necessary to succeed on the course.

In this section, we will consider both multiple mini and panel types of interview and the specific steps you will need to go through in order to prepare yourself, as well as more general interview pointers. Most of this guidance will be relevant to both types of interview and give appropriate general interview advice, but differences will be highlighted where necessary.

Multiple mini interviews

In the past, the vast majority of dental interviews have been panel-based, where two or more interviewers ask applicants a series of questions in a similar fashion to a traditional job interview. However, in recent years, a significant number of universities have moved towards the system of multiple mini interviews (MMIs), although a small number still retain the panel style of interview.

The MMI is designed to judge the suitability of a candidate to study dentistry, and is felt to give a more accurate indication of future academic performance during the course. This style of interview will have some similarities with the panel interview; however, the major difference is that applicants participate in a number of small interviews and tasks rather than just sitting in one place answering questions for the whole interview. For example, the MMI at Manchester consists of four or five seven-minute mini interviews, with interviewees having a two-minute break between stations. The format of each station will vary, but you will receive instructions explaining what you will be required to do, so ensure that you listen carefully and read any written instructions to give you a good idea of what you will be facing.

There are two main reasons for dental schools using this type of interview. Firstly, research has suggested that traditional panel interviews give a poor indication of the likely performance of the interviewee as an undergraduate; the MMI improves on this. Secondly, one of the major criticisms of the panel interview is that students can be heavily coached on the vast majority of question types and, as a result, do not give an accurate indication of their personality and character attributes at interview. MMIs are therefore specifically designed to test those attributes of the interviewee that are unlikely to be improved by participating in preparation courses. They thereby allow the dental school to build a truer picture of what each candidate is like.

Some universities are relatively tight-lipped about the exact detail of the MMI and give little information to the interviewees, while others are more open to sharing the details of exactly what will be faced.

Queen's University Belfast gives detailed exemplar material and short tutorial video clips illustrating what will be faced at each station (visit www.qub.ac.uk/schools/mdbs/Study/Medicine/HowtoApply/MMIs), whereas Bristol gives a brief paragraph outlining the basic setup:

University of Bristol

'Applicants will be assessed using an evidence-based Multiple Mini Interview (MMI) system. This is a robust and evidence-based method which has been proven to be objective and efficient. Interviewees will be assessed at a number of different "stations" covering different aspects of the skills and knowledge required to be a successful dental student and dentist.'

Source: www.bristol.ac.uk/study/undergraduate/2021/dentistry/bds-dentistry. Reprinted with kind permission from the University of Bristol *Please note that this information is relevant to the current admissions cycle. The information is reviewed each year, and may be different for the next admissions cycle, so make sure to check the university website for the most up-to-date information.*

Below are some sample MMI questions provided by www.multiplemini interview.com.

Station #1

PROMPT (Read and consider for 2 minutes):

A close friend in one of your university classes tells you that his mother was recently diagnosed with breast cancer. He feels overwhelmed by his studies and is considering dropping his courses to spend more time with his mother. How do you counsel your friend?

YOUR RESPONSE: (Speak for 8 minutes)

Station #2

PROMPT (Read and consider for 2 minutes):

Discuss one of your pastimes outside of school and how the skills you acquired will help you in your career.

YOUR RESPONSE: (Speak for 8 minutes)

Station #3:

PROMPT (Read and consider for 2 minutes):

Joe is a pizza delivery worker. The pizza shop he works for has a 30 minutes or less delivery guarantee or else the customer does not have to pay. On Joe's most recent delivery, he spots a woman bleeding on the street. There is no one else around and the woman seems to be unable to move by herself. However, Joe knows that if he returns empty handed again, he will be fired from this job which he most desperately needs. What do you think Joe should do? Justify your solution in terms of practical and ethical considerations.

YOUR RESPONSE: (Speak for 8 minutes)

Source: www.multipleminiinterview.com
Reproduced with kind permission by Astroff Consultants Inc., St Clair Avenue East, Suite 800, Toronto, Ontario, Canada M4T 2T5 at www.astroffconsultants.com

Based on these few questions, it is clear that there are a broader range of skills that need to be prepared for an MMI compared with a panel interview. Although an MMI is less formulaic than a panel interview, candidates can still take a number of steps to ensure that they are as prepared as possible, even if they might not be fully aware of what to expect until the day of the interview itself. Students should consider the following points in advance of their interview as they are the basis for the vast majority of questions.

- Communication is one of the key skills that will be assessed in the MMI, so you should therefore work on developing your ability to communicate information clearly. There are numerous ways of testing this, such as:
  - asking you to explain your interest in dentistry or your reasons for applying to the university
  - asking you to describe a picture or a painting
  - asking you to describe a series of instructions to carry out a basic task.

  In reality, any station where you are going to be speaking will be directly or indirectly assessing your ability to communicate.

  Example: You are given a picture of *Sunflowers* by Van Gogh and are asked to describe it in as much detail as possible by the interviewer.

- Communicating with different groups of people is a vital skill that dentists need. You should therefore reflect on how you might communicate effectively with different groups of people, for example children, the elderly, or individuals with disabilities. Many MMIs include role play exercises to test how effectively you can interact with people in a variety of situations. It is therefore important to be able to put into practice your thoughts on how you would communicate with different people.

  Example: You are asked to explain what factors you might need to consider when explaining a treatment plan to a patient with autism.

  Example: You are given the following scenario: You are working in a café and a customer comes to you with a complaint about the quality of her food. You need to deal with this customer and resolve her complaint.

- Practise basic manual dexterity tasks, as a number of MMIs have a section where candidates will be expected to complete some form of manual exercise. Try carrying out tasks that require repetition, focus and a steady hand as these are what the tasks are likely to be based on. To prepare for this, practise following instructions to make origami shapes, or bend wire with pliers to make shapes or patterns.

  Example: You are given a step-by-step guide to making an origami frog. You must follow the instructions to try and complete the task within three minutes.

- Practise basic observation and memory tasks. If you are shown an object for 30 seconds, can you accurately recall what it is like when it is taken away from you? If you are shown a range of objects all at once, how many can you recall a minute later?

  Example: You are given a tray of 10 objects. You must try to remember what the objects are and key details about them. When the objects are removed, you must answer questions about the things you have just seen.

- Consider your motivation for studying the course. This may be asked directly, but even if it is not, then having a clear idea of your motivation will help to guide your answers to other questions.

  Example: You are asked to explain what appeals to you about becoming a dentist.

- Make sure you understand what the key features of the university are and how the course is delivered. You may be required to explain why you are interested in studying at the university and it is this knowledge that will help you to formulate an answer.

  Example: You are asked to explain your reasons for applying to the university.

- Revisit your personal statement and reflect on key experiences in terms of work experience, leadership, teamwork, motivation, etc. You should be prepared to give evidence of how you have demonstrated that you have the skills necessary to be a dentist. Start by listing the key attributes that you think a dentist needs to master and then list at least one piece of evidence from your experiences that demonstrates you have each skill or have developed it.

Example: You are asked to explain what is meant by empathy and then asked to share an experience where you have had to demonstrate this attribute.

Example: When you were undertaking your work experience, what challenges was the dentist faced with when trying to provide high-quality care?

- Look at different methods of data presentation, for example, different styles of table and graph. Practise describing to somebody what is being shown by these graphical representations.

Example: Describe the main trends shown by this graph. Can you suggest reasons for the patterns shown.

Figure 2   Percentage of 5-year-old children with decay experience in England, 2012

Source: www.england.nhs.uk/wp-content/uploads/2014/02/
dental-info-pack.pdf

- Practise responding to situations involving ethical dilemmas in both clinical and non-clinical contexts. An understanding of the standards required of dental professionals can help you to respond appropriately to such situations. These can be found at https://standards.gdc-uk.org.

  Example: While you are treating a patient, they ask for all of their teeth to be removed and replaced with dental implants. How do you respond to this situation and what ethical issues does it raise?

- Often, interview questions can incorporate completely random elements that seem unrelated to the dental profession. These are usually designed to see what your communication skills are like and if you can stay calm in unexpectedly stressful situations.

  Example: You are asked to describe your family.

- Read the invitation to interview letter that the university has sent to you. Often this will give you more details about what to expect on the day and may drop some subtle hints about the interview process.

- Consider and practise the questions that are likely to be asked at a panel interview (see below). Although most of them probably won't come up in the MMI, they will still provide you with opportunities to hone your communication skills and reflect on your experience and motivation. This will help to improve the overall impression you make.

Panel interviews

As discussed above, the traditional panel-style interview has been phased out by a number of dental schools to be replaced by the MMI. Although this type of interview is somewhat easier to prepare for due to the well-known nature of the potential questions, it can be very easy to fall into the trap of memorising pre-rehearsed answers. The questions that are listed on pages 96–101 are designed to give you an opportunity to gather your thoughts and reflect on the various aspects of your application rather than devise set answers that you then rehearse and regurgitate in an interview.

Questions to reflect on in preparation for your interview

The questions discussed below should be considered regardless of the type of interview that you are attending. Although you will not be asked the majority of these questions in an MMI, preparing responses will help

Table 5 Typical interviews – 2020/21

University	Type of interview	Number on panel	Other information
Belfast	MMIs designed to test a range of non-cognitive skills	n/a	Scores at interview are used to rank applicants. Offers are made to the highest-ranking interviewees
Birmingham	MMIs	n/a	Circuit of 10–12 stations, approximately 1 hour in total
Bristol	MMIs	n/a	Score will be ranked and offers made to those with the highest scores
Cardiff	MMIs	n/a	12 stations in total, each station 5 minutes maximum, 2 stations are rest stations
Dundee	MMIs	n/a	Consists of 10 7-minute interviews
Glasgow	Panel	n/a	MMIs have been temporarily suspended due to Covid-19 and replaced by traditional panel
King's	MMIs	n/a	40–50 minutes in total
Leeds	MMIs	n/a	MMI lasts for about half a day
Liverpool	MMIs	n/a	None
Manchester	MMIs	n/a	4-or 5-stations. each 7 minutes long
Newcastle	Panel interview	2	The interview lasts for approximately 20 minutes
Plymouth	MMIs	n/a	7 stations, the interview lasts for approximately 50 minutes
Queen Mary	Panel interview	3	The panel can include tutors, admissions staff, dentists and current students
Sheffield	Panel interview	3	The panel comprises 2 members of academic staff and a senior dental student. The interview lasts for up to 15 minutes

you to develop a real understanding of your reasons for applying and this will shine through in subtle ways in any interview.

Question: Why did you decide to apply to this dental school?

Comment: The panel will be looking for evidence of research, and that your reasons are based on informed judgement rather than just picking a university randomly from a list. Probably the best possible answer would start with 'I came to your open day ...', because you can then proceed to tell them why you like their university so much, what impressed you about the university and facilities, and how the atmosphere of the place would particularly suit you. If you are/were unable to attend a physical open day, look for virtual events before you are interviewed so that you can show you are aware of the environment, both academic and physical, and that you like the place. If you know people who are at the dental school or university, speak to them to get firsthand feedback about their experiences.

You should also know about the course structure; the website will give detailed information. Although on the surface all dental courses appear to cover broadly the same subjects, there can be big differences between the ways in which courses are delivered and in the opportunities for patient contact, and your interviewers will expect you to know about their specific course.

Another useful source of information is the Discover Uni website (https://discoveruni.gov.uk), which gives details of student feedback about each university and each course they offer. If there are particular areas that a university scores very highly on, it may be worth mentioning as a factor that has influenced your decision.

Answers to avoid are, for example, ones such as 'Reputation' (unless you know in detail the areas for which the dental school is highly regarded), 'I don't want to move away from my friends', 'You take a lot of retake students' or 'My dad says it's easy to get a place here'.

Question: Why do you want to be a dentist?

Comment: This is the question that all interviewees expect. Given that the interviewers will be aware that you are expecting the question, they will also expect your answer to be carefully planned. If you look surprised and say something like 'Um ... well ... I haven't really thought about why ...' you can expect to be rejected. Other answers to avoid are those along the lines of 'The money' or 'It's easier than medicine'.

Many students are worried that they will sound insincere when they answer this question. The way to avoid this is to try to bring in reasons that are personal to you: for instance, an incident that sparked your interest (perhaps a visit to your own dentist), or an aspect of your work experience that particularly fascinated you. The important thing is to try to express clearly what interested you instead of generalising your answers. Rather than saying 'Dentistry combines science, working with people and the chance to have control over your career' – which says little about you – tell the interviewers about the way in which your interest progressed.

Here is an example of a carefully considered answer.

> *'I used to really enjoy going to the dentist when I was young. My dentist was brilliant at explaining things clearly and patiently, and I was interested in the technology that was being used. When I was thinking about my career, I arranged to shadow another dentist, and the more time I spent at the surgery, the more I realised that I had the skills to follow this career. It also gave me the chance to find out about what being a dentist is really like. The things that particularly interest me about dentistry are ...'*

It is vital that you do not learn this quote and repeat it at your interview. Ensure that your answer is not only personal to you, but also honest. With luck, the interviewers will pick up on something that you said about work experience and ask you more questions about this. Since 'Why do you want to be a dentist?' is such an obvious question, interviewers often try to find out the information in different ways. Expect questions such as 'When did your interest in dentistry start?' or 'What was it about your work experience that finally convinced you that dentistry was for you?' In these instances, make sure that you directly answer the question that is being asked rather than the one that you were expecting.

Question: I see that you spent two weeks with your dentist. Was there anything that surprised you?

Comment: Variations on this question could include 'Was there anything that particularly interested you?', 'Was there anything you found off-putting?' or simply 'Tell me about your work experience'. What these questions really mean is: 'Are you able to show us that you were interested in what was happening during your work experience?'

Returning to the original question, answering either 'Yes' or 'No' without explanation will not gain you many marks. Similarly, saying 'Yes, I was surprised by the number of patients who seemed very scared' says nothing about your awareness of the dentist's approach to their patients. However, answering: 'Yes, I was surprised by the number of patients who seemed very scared. What struck me, however, was the way in which the dentist dealt with each patient as an individual, sometimes being sympathetic, sometimes explaining things in great detail and sometimes using humour to relax them. For instance ...' shows that you were interested enough to be aware of more than the most obvious things.

Sentences that start with 'For example ...' and 'For instance ...' are particularly important, as they allow you to demonstrate your interest.

As previously mentioned in Chapter 2, you should keep a diary of things that you saw during your work experience so that you do not forget and can provide examples. You should then review your diary before interview to refresh your memory.

Question: Can you tell me about something that you have read recently in relation to dentistry?

Comment: If you are interested in making dentistry your career, the selectors will expect you to be interested enough in the subject to want to read about it. Some good sources of information that you may want to make use of are the GDC website (www.gdc-uk.org), www.dentistry. co.uk, the BBC news website and broadsheet newspapers. You should get into the habit of checking the news every day to see if there are any dentistry-related stories. You should not just rely on things that you read years ago; however, you may have followed a particular issue for a number of years, and it is totally appropriate in this situation to revisit historical items in order to give depth to something you have read more recently.

Question: During your work experience, you had the chance to discuss dentistry with the practitioner. What do you know about the way NHS dentists are paid?

Comment: You must be aware of the nuts and bolts of running a dental practice; in particular, it is worth understanding the difference between NHS and private work and the way in which the NHS is funded. You should also have an idea about what a dentist earns and what proportion of it goes back into running the practice. Similar questions might focus on how much dentists are paid for different types of treatment, or how much NHS patients pay for treatment.

Question: Should dental treatment be free on the NHS?

Comment: Although not specifically about dentistry, this type of question can be useful for an admissions tutor to see how you can think on your feet about wider issues. Obviously this type of question needs you to understand what the issues surrounding the NHS are and to have knowledge of what is going on in the world; but more importantly, it needs you to be able to form and express arguments and opinions. If you are struggling to figure out exactly how to respond to such a question, it is worth taking a moment to gather your thoughts before you reply. It is also worth considering both sides of the argument and expressing your reflection on these, as it shows that you have an appreciation of the range of issues involved.

Question: What qualities should a dentist possess?

Comment: Don't simply list the qualities. The interviewer hasn't asked the question because the interviewer is puzzled about what these qualities are; they have asked it to give you a chance to show that you are aware of them, and that you possess them. The best way to answer this is to use phrases such as 'During my work experience at the Smith and Smith Dental Practice, I was able to observe/talk to the dentist, and I became aware that …', or 'Communication is very important: for instance, when I was shadowing my dentist, there was a patient who …' Always try to relate these general questions to your own experiences.

Question: Do you know what periodontics is?

Comment: It is highly unlikely that you will be asked specific questions in relation to the technical aspects of dentistry as you haven't yet studied the subject. However, something you have written in your personal statement or mentioned in one of your responses might move the conversation in this direction. This provides another good reason for carrying out careful research into the field of dentistry before applying and for asking questions during work experience. Remember that when you are asked this type of question, the interviewer is not expecting you to have an encyclopaedic knowledge of the area, but is interested in seeing whether you have a solid basic knowledge. It would be worth starting your answer with a basic definition and then, if you have further knowledge or experience of the area, expanding on it. It may also provide another opportunity to discuss a relevant article or current issue that you have seen or to further discuss an experience from a work placement.

If you have absolutely no idea about what is being asked, try first to think about whether you have any reference points that might enable you to make an educated guess; in this situation it is preferable to discuss your ideas and to show the interviewers your thought processes than to just stay silent and refuse to answer. There are times when an interviewer will purposely ask a question that is difficult just so they can see how you respond under pressure and if you can think on your feet.

Question: Dentistry requires a high degree of manual dexterity. How have you developed this skill?

Comment: The question about manual dexterity is very interesting and often ignored by candidates. Manual dexterity means being able to perform intricate tasks with your hands. Dentists have to work in a confined and sensitive area (the mouth) using precision instruments, in situations where accuracy is vital and where there is little margin for error. If you have trouble picking up a coffee cup without knocking it over or if you always press the wrong keys when you work on a computer, dentistry may not be the best career for you. The interviewers will need to be reassured that you have the manual skills to be able to work on other people's teeth. Good examples of tasks that require a high degree of manual dexterity include sewing, embroidery, model-making and playing a musical instrument.

Manual dexterity is a very important factor that should not be overlooked in the selection process. Students, professionals and admissions tutors to whom I've spoken have all indicated that without this quality a prospective candidate might as well not continue with his or her application. If you are not able to give an example of your own skills, take up a hobby that involves precision work, before it is too late. Admissions tutors don't want students bringing examples of their handiwork to interview, but you do need be able to discuss any relevant experiences.

Whatever you do, do not lie about the examples of manual dexterity that you provide. One admissions tutor tells the story of a young man who claimed that he liked icing cakes in his spare time. He brought in photographs of some of the cakes he had iced but it became clear, after very little questioning, that it was his mother who had actually done the work. This did not go down well with the panel, as you can imagine!

Question: How do you cope with stress?

Comment: Dentistry can be a stressful occupation. Dentists have to deal with difficult people, those who are scared and those who react badly when in a dental surgery. Furthermore, there are few 'standard' situations: everyone's mouth and teeth are different, as are their problems, and things can go wrong. In these circumstances, the dentist cannot panic but must remain calm and rational. In addition, the nature of the profession means that the financial aspects of running a business may also be a source of stress. The interviewers want to make a judgement as to whether you will be able to cope with the demands that the course and the job throw up. Once again, be sincere. Reflect on a particularly stressful time in your life and how you have coped through it. Remember, it is always best to use experiences from your own life than to talk generally.

Question: I see that you enjoy reading. What is the most recent book that you have read?

Comment: Although it may sound obvious, if you have written that you enjoy reading on your UCAS application, make sure that you have actually read something recently. Admissions tutors will be able to tell you stories about interviewees who look at them with absolute surprise when they are asked about books, despite reading featuring in the personal statement. Answers such as 'Well ... I haven't had much time recently, but ... let me see ... I read *Top Gear* magazine last month, and ... oh yes ... I had to read *Jane Eyre* for my English GCSE' will not help your chances. The same advice is also true for any other interests you put on your personal statement: if you put it down, you need to be prepared to talk about it!

Question: What interests do you have?

Comment: Don't say 'Watch TV' or 'Go shopping'. Mention something that involves working or communicating with others, for instance sport or music. Use the question to demonstrate that you possess the qualities required in a dentist. However, don't make your answer so insincere that the interviewers realise that you are trying to impress them. Saying 'I relax most effectively when I go to the local dental surgery to shadow the dentist' will not convince them.

Other questions to consider

Remember that you will have only limited time in an interview and as a result will only be asked a relatively modest number of questions. There is therefore no chance of you being asked all of the questions listed below, but preparing as widely as possible will help to increase your all-round knowledge and skills, which will come across at any interview you attend.

- Why do you want to be a dentist?
- What have you done to investigate dentistry?
- Give me an example of how you cope with stress.
- Why did you apply to this dental school?
- During your work experience, did anything surprise you?
- During your work experience, did anything shock you?
- Tell me about preventive dentistry.
- If you had to organise a campaign to improve oral health, how would you go about it?
- What role do dentists play in improving oral health?
- Why do dentists recommend the fluoridation of water supplies?
- There has been a good deal of negative publicity about mercury fillings. Do you think that they are dangerous?
- What is gingivitis?
- How are NHS dentists funded?
- Have you read any articles about dentistry recently?
- What advances can we expect in dental technology/treatment in the future?
- What have you done to demonstrate your commitment to the community?
- What would you contribute to this dental school?
- What are your best/worst qualities?
- What was the last novel that you read? Did you like it?
- What do you do to relax?
- What is your favourite A level subject?
- Do dentists treat children differently from adults?
- What precautions need to be taken with patients who are HIV positive?
- What is the role of the dental nurse/technician?
- How does teamwork apply to the role of a dentist?
- What role does a dentist have in diagnosing other medical problems?

How to succeed in the interview

You should prepare for both types of interview as if you are preparing for an examination. Start by revisiting your personal statement as this can be a common starting point for interviewers when thinking about questions to ask you. In particular, revisit the details of your work experience so that you can recount details of your time with a dentist and reflect on the key experiences you had and lessons you learned. Then look through articles you have saved from the newspaper, the internet and magazines in relation to dentistry, and consider all the things that you have mentioned in your personal statement. It is vital that you are truthful in your personal statement, as it is very easy to get caught out if you have lied.

When you are preparing for an interview, try to have at least one mock interview so that you can get some feedback on your answers. Your school may be able to help you. If not, there are many providers that offer a mock interview service. Friends of your parents may also be able to help. As mentioned previously, do not memorise set answers to questions; this is very easy to spot during an interview and will make you seem insincere. It is much better to have a good idea of roughly what you want to say and then put it across in a natural way. If possible, video your mock interview so that you are aware of the way you come across in such a situation.

At the end of your interview

In a panel situation you may be given the opportunity to ask a question at the end, although this won't happen in an MMI. Bear in mind that the interviews are carefully timed, and that your attempts to impress the panel with 'clever' questions may do quite the opposite. The golden rule is: only ask a question if you are genuinely interested in the answer (which, of course, is one you were unable to find the answer to on the website or when speaking to other people during your visit). Remember that the people interviewing you have lots to do and very little time to do it in, so most questions are better off asked to staff or current students that you meet at other points on the day of your interview.

Questions to avoid

- What is the structure of the first year of the course?
- Will I be able to live in a hall of residence?
- When will I first have contact with patients?

As well as being boring questions, the answers to these will be available in the prospectus. If you need to ask these questions, it will be obvious to your interviewers that you have not done any serious research.

Remember: if in doubt, don't ask a question. End by saying: 'All of my questions have been answered by the prospectus and the students who showed me around the dental school. Thank you very much for an interesting day.' Smile, shake hands (if appropriate) and say goodbye.

General interview tips

As in any interview, appearance and body language are just as important as the answers you give to the questions you are being asked. The impression that you create can have a big impact. Remember that if the interviewers cannot picture you as a dentist in the future, they are unlikely to offer you a place.

Body language

- Make eye contact with the interviewers, but don't stare at them!
- When you say hello to the interviewer, remember to smile.
- Sit up straight, but adopt a position that you feel comfortable in.
- Don't wave your hands around too much, but don't keep them gripped together to stop them moving either. Fold them across your lap, or rest them on the arms of the chair.
- Avoid annoying and repetitive body movements, such as jiggling your leg or tapping the table.

Speech

- Talk at your normal pace and beware of speaking too quickly. When you are nervous it is very easy to speed up your speech, so make a conscious effort to slow down if needed.
- Don't use slang or offensive language.
- Avoid saying 'Erm …', 'You know', 'Sort of' and 'Like'. These are often put into sentences without really realising; another good reason to have mock interviews so that these habits can be highlighted to you.
- Say 'Hello' at the start of the interview, and thank the interviewer(s) and say 'Goodbye' at the end.

Dress and appearance

- Wear clothes that show you have made an effort for the interview. In reality, this should mean formal, smart dress. If you are unsure, it is better to be overdressed than to be underdressed with no way of making yourself look smarter.
- Make sure that you are clean and tidy.
- Avoid using overpowering perfume or aftershave.
- Clean your nails and shoes.

- Wash your hair.
- Avoid excessive piercings.

How you are selected

During the interview, the interviewers (both MMI and panel) will be assessing you in various categories. Each interviewer follows careful guidelines to mark your performance so that they can compare each candidate fairly.

The scoring system will vary from university to university, but you are likely to be scored in a number of categories, with the dental school setting a minimum mark that you will have to gain if you are to be made an offer. For example, Bristol University gives the following information about the scoring of its MMI interview.

University of Bristol

'Applicants' performance at the MMIs is scored by assessors and ranked by the Admissions Office. Those candidates with the strongest overall performance receive offers.'

Source: www.bristol.ac.uk/study/undergraduate/2021/dentistry/bds-dentistry
Reprinted with kind permission from the University of Bristol
Please note that this information is relevant to the current admissions cycle. The information is reviewed each year, and may be different for the next admissions cycle, so make sure to check the university website for the most up-to-date information.

If you are below the cut-off score but close to it, you may be put on an official or unofficial waiting list. If you are offered a place, you will receive a letter from the dental school telling you what you need to achieve in your A levels: this is called a conditional offer. In addition, the conditions of your offer will be added to UCAS Track, although this can take some time, so don't worry if you are made to wait a while after initially hearing from the university. Post-A level students who have achieved the necessary grades may be given unconditional offers in terms of the academic requirements, but may still be made conditional offers in relation to criminal record and health checks. If you are unlucky, all you will get is a notification from UCAS saying that you have been rejected. If this happens, it is not necessarily the end of the road in dentistry, as you may be able to reapply as a post-A level applicant. What you must do in this situation is contact the universities that you applied to and ask for feedback about why you were unsuccessful. Some universities will be more helpful than others and give relatively detailed feedback, which will give you points to consider. However, be warned, some universities don't give feedback, while others will just send a standard letter with no details about your particular application.

What happens next?

When UCAS has received replies from all of your choices you will then have about a month to make up your mind about where you want to go. If you have only one offer, you have two choices. One is to accept the choice and aim to get the grades to go to that university; the other is to reject the choice, if you have decided for whatever reason that you don't want to go to that university. If you choose to go down the latter route, you must then apply either the following year or add additional choices through what is known as UCAS Extra, although it is highly unlikely at this point in time that places for dentistry will appear on Extra.

If you have more than one offer, you have to accept one as your firm choice, and may accept another as your insurance choice. If the place where you really want to study makes a lower offer than one of your other choices, do not be tempted to choose the lower offer as your insurance choice since you are obliged to go to the dental school that you have put as your firm choice if you achieve the necessary grades. If you narrowly miss the grades required by your firm offer, you may still be accepted on the course. You would have to accept this offer so you would not be able to go to your insurance choice. You can go to your insurance choice only if your firm choice will not accept you. So, if you had put the dental school you really wanted to study at as your insurance choice, in this instance you would not be able to accept a place there.

If you are unsuccessful, there remains the option of completing a first degree and then attempting graduate entry or studying dentistry overseas (see page 130).

Current issues in dentistry

As part of your research into dentistry and during your work experience, you will probably come across news and other relevant articles about a range of current issues related to the profession. While an awareness of what is going on in the world of dentistry may not be of any use in choosing which dental school to apply to, it is absolutely essential when it comes to your preparation for interview, as you will be expected to have a solid understanding of such issues. The aim of this section, therefore, is to give you an idea of some of these issues and provide a starting point for you to do further research. While you are reading and researching, it is important once again to keep a notebook to hand so that you can jot down anything of interest; your notes will then be the perfect starting point for your revision when you receive notice of your first interview. There is a wealth of information relating to the world of dentistry, but, in my experience, sites like www.dentistry.co.uk, www.bda.org, www.dentalhealth.org and www.bbc.co.uk are worth checking frequently to keep abreast of important developments.

Covid-19

A global pandemic of the Covid-19 virus was declared in early 2020, and a UK lockdown followed in March 2020. This immediately had a significant impact on the provision of dental care across the UK.

Due to the proximity that dentists have to their patients when undertaking routine check-ups and treatment, there is a high risk to those providing (and receiving) this type of care. The Covid-19 guidance from the NHS and Public Health England for operating as a dentist is therefore highly detailed and requires a great deal of planning and preparation to ensure that the patient and dental team are safe. Some of the measures include the provision and enhanced use of Personal Protective Equipment (PPE), the use of remote initial consultations and enhanced cleaning of facilities between patients. Full details can be found at www.england.nhs.uk/coronavirus/wp-content/uploads/sites/52/2020/06/C1029-SOP-Transition-to-recovery-A-phased-transition-for-dental-practices-towards-the-resumption-of-the-full-r.pdf..

During the pandemic, statistics have shown that there have been millions of missed appointments across the country, with a large reduction in the number of referrals for oral cancer investigations. These facts, coupled with a reported increase in snacking habits during lockdown periods, are likely to have far-reaching consequences in terms of the oral health of the general population.

Sugar tax on soft drinks

In 2016, the government announced plans for a sugar tax to be introduced on soft drinks depending on the quantity of sugar in the drink. This tax came into force in April 2018 and is currently levied at the rate of 18p per litre on drinks with more than 5g of sugar per 100ml and 24p per litre on drinks with more than 8g per 100ml.

In the lead-up to the implementation of the tax, many of the leading soft-drink manufacturers altered the recipes of the products that would be affected in order to lower sugar levels. Brands such as Fanta, Lucozade, Vimto and Ribena have already made significant and noticeable reductions. However, not all sugary drinks are included in the tax. Notable exceptions are pure fruit juices (as extra sugar isn't added) and drinks that contain at least 75% milk (due to the benefits of calcium).

Table 6 Examples of drinks with reduced sugar content

Drink	Original sugar content (g per 100ml)	New sugar content (g per 100ml)
Im Bru	10.3	4.7
Lucozade	13	4.5
Ribena	10	Less than 4.5

When the idea was initially proposed, it was expected that it would raise approximately £500 million per year in tax receipts, however, due to the steps taken by manufacturers, this figure has been revised down to approximately £240 million. The supporters of the tax have used this information to point to the success that there has already been in driving down sugar content in drinks.

Similar types of tax across the globe have had some success in reducing consumption of fizzy drinks. For example, Mexico introduced a 10% sugar tax in 2014. Within the first year, there was a 12% reduction in fizzy drink sales. There is no doubt that this type of tax has the potential to have a massive effect on oral health, but only time will tell as to whether there is a significant impact in the UK.

The nation's oral health

There has been a steady improvement in oral health in the UK in recent decades due to a number of factors, including:

- developments in dental treatment
- provision of preventive and restorative dental treatment
- increased awareness of dental health
- fluoridation of water
- fluoride in toothpaste.

There has been a significant push by organisations such as the British Dental Health Foundation to raise public awareness of the need for good general oral health. This has been achieved by carrying out educational campaigns such as National Smile Month and providing information to the public regarding issues such as mouth cancer and fluoridation. It is important to recognise the shift from talking about good dental health to talking about good oral health: this represents the fact that it is the health not just of the teeth but of the whole mouth that is important. Promoting the virtues of good oral health in this way continues to have a significant impact on levels of public awareness.

The National Institute for Health and Clinical Excellence (NICE) publishes guidelines on the frequency of dental check-ups, with the recommended interval between check-ups being the same (usually six months) regardless of the patient's age and oral health, but official NHS guidance is:

> 'You may assume you should have a dental check-up every 6 months, but some people may not need to go so often and others may need more frequent checks. Your dentist will suggest when you should have your next check-up based on how good your oral health is. The time between check-ups can vary from 3 months to 2 years, depending on how healthy your teeth and gums are and your risk of future problems.'

Source: www.nhs.uk/live-well/healthy-body/dental-check-ups

In spite of the progress and advances made in recent decades, there is still much work to do to further improve oral health. This can be effectively illustrated by scrutinising some of the statistics provided by the Oral Health Foundation for National Smile Month 2020 (www.dental health.org/oral-health-statistics). Before looking at these figures, it is worth taking a guess at what you think the actual values are – you may be shocked by some of the statistics that are presented.

What do you think the figures are for the following?

- The number of school days on average that are missed per pupil due to dental problems.
- The percentage of adults that don't go to the dentist regularly.
- The percentage of adults with visible plaque.
- The percentage of adults that do not brush twice a day with a fluoride toothpaste.
- The percentage of adults that have had at least one tooth extracted.

The answers are as follows.

- Number of school days missed: 3.
- Adults that don't go to the dentist regularly: 39%.
- Adults with visible plaque: 66%.
- Adults that do not brush twice a day: 25%.
- Adults that have had at least one tooth extracted: 74%.

These statistics paint a sobering picture of the state of the nation's teeth, and any oral health professional would agree that there is still much work to do to educate people about maintaining good oral health.

Children's oral health

Every 10 years, an extensive national survey is conducted regarding the oral health of children. The 2013 survey results, published in 2015, revealed that although there was a reduction in the 'extent and severity' of tooth decay in the permanent teeth of 12–15-year-olds between 2003 and 2013, a large percentage of children continue to be affected by tooth decay. (Source: https://digital.nhs.uk/data-and-information/areas-of-interest/public-health/children-s-dental-health-survey.)

There is no doubt that concerns regarding the oral health of children stem from the high levels of sugar in their diet. One of the major contributing factors towards tooth decay and erosion in children is the consumption of fizzy drinks; children who drink several fizzy drinks a day massively increase the chance of damage occurring to their teeth.

The biennial survey of the oral health of five-year-old children (https://assets.publishing.service.gov.uk/government/uploads/system/uploads/attachment_data/file/873492/NDEP_for_England_OH_Survey_5yr_2019_v1.0.pdf) revealed some interesting facts. The main finding was that, in 2019, 23.4% of five-year-olds in England had some dental decay. In spite of the progress made with children's oral health in recent decades, this figure has increased from 23.3% in 2017 and is still a shocking statistic. As a consequence, it is a certainty that improving the oral health of young children will continue to be a hot topic. There is also no doubt that the success of the sugar tax in improving these statistics will be scrutinised carefully in years to come.

Mouth cancer

What is mouth cancer?

Mouth cancer is historically thought of as a disease affecting mainly older males; however, over recent years, the incidence in women and children has significantly increased. One of the major issues with mouth cancer is that there is poor public awareness of the disease and its symptoms. Mouth cancer can affect any part of the mouth, including the lips, tongue, cheeks and throat, and has a number of characteristic symptoms, including ulcers that do not heal within three weeks, red and white patches or unusual lumps or swellings in the mouth. A major problem with being able to diagnose and treat mouth cancer is that many people displaying symptoms will ignore them for a long time, thereby delaying effective treatment.

What role do dentists play in relation to mouth cancer?

Early detection of mouth cancer is one of the key factors in successful treatment, a message that is reinforced by the annual Mouth Cancer Action Month campaign (www.mouthcancer.org). This means that regular screening by dentists plays a vital role in the process of diagnosing and treating those with the disease. This further supports the idea that dentists are responsible not just for treating teeth; they are in fact involved in every aspect of oral health.

What is the incidence of mouth cancer?

According to Cancer Research UK, between 2015 and 2017, there were some 12,200 new cases of head and neck cancer diagnosed per year. Head and neck cancer includes all forms of cancer found in the mouth, the nasal cavities and the larynx. Worryingly, the incidence of the disease has increased 33% since the early 1990s.

Who is at risk?

There are a number of risk factors associated with mouth cancer. However, chewing tobacco or another similar product is the main risk, with excessive alcohol consumption, poor diet and the human papilloma virus (HPV) also being contributing factors. Smoking and drinking to excess is a particular problem because alcohol can aid tobacco absorption in the mouth. This can increase the risk up to thirtyfold.

Antibiotic resistance

Antibiotic resistance is the ability of pathogenic bacteria to resist the action of antibiotics, and it continues to be a major threat to all areas of medicine, including dentistry. Resistance is driven by the overuse and over-prescription of these drugs, both to humans and in agriculture, and in the long term has the potential to render all currently known antibiotics useless.

It is unclear what the future holds in relation to the use of antibiotics, but there is consensus that unless new drugs are discovered or alternative methods of treatment are developed, there will be a massive impact on our ability to successfully treat common infections and carry out invasive treatments that rely on the use of antibiotics.

Tooth whitening regulation

In recent years, there has been a large increase in the number of unregulated tooth whitening treatments administered to the general public. Thousands of people each year have this type of treatment carried out in beauty salons, shopping centres and high streets by individuals with no formal training in tooth whitening. A large increase in the number of complaints made against such companies has led the GDC to call for tooth whitening treatments to be more tightly regulated. The position of the GDC is now that any sort of cosmetic intervention to improve the whiteness of teeth is considered to be a dental treatment and as such should only be administered by a dentist or other regulated dental professional, such as a hygienist. It is therefore illegal for an organisation to carry out tooth whitening if there is not a suitably qualified dental professional present. Home whitening kits are still available, but because of the potential risks involved, they are also considered to be potentially dangerous and should be avoided.

The law currently states that tooth-whitening products containing between 0.1%–6% hydrogen peroxide should not be made directly available to the consumer and can only be administered by a dental professional to a patient over 18 years of age. Any products with greater than 6% hydrogen peroxide are illegal and anything containing under 0.1% can be sold directly to the consumer.

Tooth whitening is often carried out to improve the appearance of teeth if staining has occurred due to smoking, drinking tea, coffee and red wine, or just due to age. Common treatments involve using a bleaching gel to make this improvement, but if incorrectly done, this can result in problems such as removing the enamel from teeth and causing gum damage, hence why only qualified dental professionals can carry out treatments of this type.

The recent history of NHS dentistry in England

The history of NHS dentistry in the last decade is complex and to fully understand the current landscape, it is necessary to go back to the sweeping reforms of 2006 as a starting point.

What were the 2006 reforms?

In April 2006, the government carried out sweeping reforms of the system, which were heralded as a new dawn for NHS dentistry and were designed to entice more dentists into the service, thereby improving access to dental care. Under the old system, dentists were paid for each treatment they performed (there were around 400 separate charges), whereas the current system gives dentists a guaranteed income for providing a certain number of courses of NHS treatment to any patient requiring care. The reforms also targeted the pricing system and simplified the structure into three bands as follows:

- **Band 1:** covers an examination, diagnosis and advice. If necessary, it also includes X-rays, a scale and polish and planning for further treatment.
- **Band 2:** covers all treatment covered by Band 1, plus additional treatment, such as fillings, root canal treatment and removing teeth (extractions).
- **Band 3:** covers all treatment covered by Bands 1 and 2, plus more complex procedures, such as crowns, dentures and bridges.

Source: www.nhs.uk/common-health-questions/dental-health/what-is-included-in-each-nhs-dental-band-charge

Note that in this system, only one dental charge is incurred even if you need to visit more than once to complete a course of dental treatment. If you need more treatment at the same charge level (e.g. an additional filling) within two months of seeing your dentist, this is also free of charge.

The box below shows a more detailed breakdown of different costs as they stand at this point in time. Although the costs have changed over the past 14 years, the general structure of charges remains the same. You will see that all of the procedures listed fit into one of the three bands. A person pays only once – one charge for each course of treatment. For example, for a check-up, X-ray, teeth polish, a simple filling and a crown, a patient would pay a total of £269.30 if they all occurred within a two-month period. This pricing structure was designed to try to bring an end to the so-called 'drill and fill' culture and allow dentists to spend more time promoting preventive dentistry.

Dental procedure costs

Band 1 dental treatment: £22.70

This covers one or more treatments (as many as are necessary) from the following:

- adjusting false teeth (dentures) or orthodontic appliances, such as braces
- applying sealants or fluoride preparations to the surfaces of your teeth
- a clinical examination, assessment and report
- marginal correction of fillings
- moulds of your teeth – for example, to see how your teeth bite together
- an orthodontic assessment and report
- a scale and polish (if clinically necessary)
- coloured photographs
- taking a sample of cells or tissue from your mouth for examination
- treating sensitive cementum (the tissue that covers the root of a tooth)
- X-rays
- Emergency treatment (when you need to see a dentist immediately).

Band 2 dental treatment: £62.10

This can cover anything listed in band 1 above, plus any of the following:

- an addition to your dentures – such as adding a clasp or a tooth
- apicectomy – removing the tip of the root of a tooth
- a mouth guard to correct your 'bite' (doesn't include a laboratory-made appliance)
- fillings
- free gingival grafts – when healthy tissue from the roof of your mouth is attached to your teeth where the root is exposed
- frenectomy or frenotomy – surgery to the folds of tissue that connect your tongue, lips and cheeks to your jaw bone
- treatment for severe form of gum disease – such as root planing (cleaning bacteria from the roots of your teeth),deep scaling and a polish, or a gingivectomy (removal of gum tissue)
- oral surgery – such as removing a cyst, or soft tissue surgery to the mouth or lips
- pulpotomy – removing dental pulp (the soft tissue at the centre of a tooth)
- relining and rebasing dentures
- removing teeth (extraction)
- root canal treatment
- sealant to fill small holes and seal any grooves in your teeth
- splinting loose teeth – for example, after an accident (this doesn't include laboratory-made splints)
- transplanting teeth.

Band 3 dental treatment: £269.30

This can cover anything listed in bands 1 and 2 above, plus any of the following:

- bridges – a fixed replacement for a missing tooth or teeth
- crowns – a type of cap that completely covers your real tooth
- dentures
- inlays, pinlays and onlays – used to restore damaged teeth
- orthodontic treatment and appliances such as braces (clinical, not cosmetic)
- other custom-made appliances, not including sports guards
- veneers and palatal veneers – new surfaces for the front or back of a tooth (clinical, not cosmetic).

Source: www.nhs.uk/common-health-questions/dental-health/what-is-included-in-each-nhs-dental-band-charge

Reprinted with kind permission from NHS Choices

How were the reforms received?

When the reforms were introduced, many patients welcomed the changes because they felt they would go some way to resolving certain problems associated with accessing NHS dental care, in addition to making the pricing structure clearer. However, the changes did mean that the cost of some basic treatments increased.

Practising dentists were more sceptical of the reforms: a survey of dentists carried out by the BDA in the wake of the changes revealed that 55% of dentists did not think that they allowed them to see more patients. Before the reforms, according to the BDA, 32% of dentists performed 95% of their work on NHS patients, but this fell to 25% of dentists since the reforms. The reforms led to more than 1,000 dentists walking away from NHS work.

What was the impact of the reforms?

On the whole, the impact of the reforms was initially perceived to be negative, with a number of statistics and comments backing this up. Perhaps the most damning statistic that came to light following the reforms was that, in the two years following their introduction, 1 million fewer patients visited an NHS dentist. In addition to this, according to the BDA, 85% of dentists did not feel that the reforms had improved access. A report from the House of Commons Health Committee also stated that the reforms had not solved the 'fundamental problems'. It had also been implied that some dentists were less inclined to perform more complex treatments such as crowns and bridges because they received less money for them.

The BDA said the reforms did not give dentists enough time to do preventive work. This caused strong feelings among dentists, so much so that in some areas up to three-quarters of dentists threatened to quit the NHS. According to the BDA, the deal meant that dentists had to carry out 95% of the courses of treatment which they previously did to get the same money, thus leaving little time for addressing the causes of poor oral health. One of the key issues was that some dentists 'used up' the number of courses they had been allocated prior to the end of the year. This ultimately meant that they had to turn away any extra patients as they had been given no further funding to treat them.

In spite of some of the negative feelings about the NHS dental reforms, it is important to consider the statistics in terms of patient care: in the 24-month period ending in June 2013, 2.8 million more patients had been seen by a dentist than at the historic low point in June 2008. Although this does not tell the whole story about the reservations that dentists had about the reforms, it does indicate that they were successful in increasing patient contact and so the reforms should in some lights be seen as having an overall positive impact.

The 2009 review

In 2009, an independent review of NHS dental services was published that made recommendations about the way forward for dental care in this country. Professor Jimmy Steele, Professor of Oral Health Services Research at Newcastle University, engaged with dental professionals, NHS staff, patients and patient representative groups to compile this review. One of the key changes proposed in the review was that the income of dentists was to be determined by three factors – patient list size, quality of care, and the number of courses of treatment rather than just carrying out a set number of courses. In addition to this, the report suggested that patients needed to be provided with better information about available NHS dentists and that the three-band pricing structure should be widened to 10 bands.

Following the publication of this report, the government accepted the recommendations 'in principle' and the Department of Health began to pilot them from 2011. The pilot has aimed to focus on providing the treatment that the patient needs and avoiding unnecessary interventions as well as increasing access to dental services and focusing on the oral health of children. In 2014, the findings of the pilot were published (https://assets.publishing.service.gov.uk/government/uploads/system/uploads/attachment_data/file/282760/Dental_contract_pilots_evidence_and_learning_report.pdf).

In January 2015, the findings of the pilot were used to propose a series of prototype contracts to be trialled as the next stage of the reform process. By 2020, the government had 99 dental practices and three community dental services taking part in the Dental Contract Reform Programme, although a national roll-out was yet to be decided upon.

The pace of reform continues to be very slow. This seems to be a deliberate strategy to ensure that the new system is tried, tested and fit for purpose. Lord Howe, who wrote the foreword to the document, said the following:

'I know that there has been frustration at the pace of reform. I understand this frustration but I hope there is understanding of why we have taken a measured approach. The reform we are proposing is ground breaking and, we believe, will enable primary dental services to best meet the changing oral health needs of the population.'

Fluoridation

Perhaps one of the biggest issues in dentistry in recent decades has been the fluoridation of water supplies and the impact it has on oral health. Although this issue has been around for a long time, it is still vital that you understand what the background is to the debate and the arguments for and against fluoridation.

What is fluoride?

Fluorine is a naturally occurring gas. When fluorine forms a binary compound with another element, this is known as a fluoride. Fluoride ions are found in soil, fresh water and seawater, plants and many foods.

How does fluoride work?

Fluoride is beneficial to both developing and developed teeth, as it decreases the risk of decay. Dental decay is caused by acids produced by the plaque on our teeth, which react with the sugars and other carbohydrates we eat. The acids attack the tooth enamel, which, after repeated attacks, will break down, allowing cavities to form. Fluoride acts by bonding to the tooth enamel, thereby reducing the solubility of the enamel in the acids. Fluoride also inhibits the growth of the bacteria responsible for tooth decay. There is also evidence that it helps repair the very earliest stages of decay by promoting the remineralisation of the tooth enamel. However, fluoride is not a cure-all and the risk of tooth decay can still be increased by other factors such as exposed roots, frequent sugar and carbohydrate consumption, poor oral hygiene and reduced salivary flow.

What is fluoridation?

Fluoride occurs naturally in our water supply at varying levels, usually below 1 part per million (ppm). Fluoridation is the process by which the amount of fluoride is adjusted to the optimum level that protects against tooth decay. Where fluoride is added, the natural level is increased to approximately 1 ppm.

What are the benefits of fluoridation?

Initially, the main beneficiaries of fluoridated water supplies were thought to be children under the age of five years. In areas where the concentration of fluoride in water supplies is 1 ppm, rates of decay and tooth loss in children are greatly reduced. High levels of tooth decay in children are generally associated with areas of social deprivation. This is a pattern repeated throughout the EU and the USA. The best dental health regions in the UK are the West Midlands, an area where over two-thirds of the population receive fluoridated water, and south-east England, which is predominantly an affluent area. The worst areas for dental health are those associated with higher levels of social deprivation, such as north-west England. Children living in socially deprived areas with non-fluoridated water supplies can suffer up to six times more tooth decay than those living in more affluent areas or those receiving fluoridated water supplies. For example, in the poorest communities of north-west England, as many as one in three children of pre-school age have had a general anaesthetic for tooth extraction, and in Glasgow tooth extraction is the most common reason for general anaesthesia for children under the age of 10.

Research has shown that it is not only children who benefit from fluoridated water supplies but people of all ages, as the effect of fluoride on the surface of fully developed teeth is thought to be even more important. Elderly people in particular can benefit from drinking fluoridated water. The decrease in salivary flow with age, combined with reduced manual dexterity, means that it is more difficult to keep your teeth clean as you get older. So older people are more prone to root surface decay, which is difficult to treat. As fluoride strengthens adult tooth enamel, it helps reduce the incidence of this type of decay.

It is estimated that the NHS could save approximately £4 million per year on removal of rotten teeth in hospitals if fluoridation was extended to areas around the country with particularly high levels of tooth decay; this gives a potential economic benefit to fluoridation in addition to the benefits to oral health outlined above.

Probably the two most important advantages of fluoridated water supplies, as opposed to any other method of combating tooth decay, are that it is cost-effective and, more importantly, all members of the community are reached, regardless of income, education or access to dental care.

What are the problems with fluoridation?

The only proven side-effect of drinking fluoridated water is dental fluorosis. This is mottling of the teeth caused by a disruption of the enamel formation while the teeth are developing under the gums. It occurs between birth and the age of five years, when the enamel is developing. In mild cases, dental fluorosis is purely a minor cosmetic problem, which is barely visible to either the individual or the observer. It is also thought that mild dental fluorosis may further increase the resistance of the tooth enamel to decay. In moderate to severe cases of dental fluorosis, the colouring of the teeth is very pronounced and irregularities develop on the tooth surface. Whether this is purely a cosmetic problem or whether it adversely affects the function of the teeth is a matter of some debate.

Some research has claimed links between fluorosis and higher instances of bone cancer, osteoarthritis and fractures. However, numerous studies have concluded that there is no clear evidence that fluoridation of water at the recommended level of 1mg of fluoride to every litre of water causes harm to health, apart from dental fluorosis.

Other concerns expressed about fluoridation are its effect on the environment, particularly on plants. Fluorides have been used in some pesticides and insecticides and their use is now restricted. Other industrial fluorides are one of the main pollutants in waterways and the atmosphere.

What are the ethical issues involved in fluoridation?

One of the main ethical issues with fluoridation of water supplies involves infringement of personal liberty, as it effectively medicates everyone without an individual having the choice to refuse. We have no choice over our drinking water supply other than through our water company, unless we opt to buy bottled water, the cost of which would be prohibitive for certain sections of the community.

The issue of adding fluoride remains an emotive topic, as demonstrated when the decision was made to fluoridate the water supply of Southampton in 2008. The local health authority decided to introduce fluoridation in an attempt to reduce levels of tooth decay in the city. This plan was carried out in spite of a public consultation that suggested that 72% of 10,000 local people were opposed to the plan. As a result, local residents mounted a legal challenge, which had the backing of local politicians. Their opposition was based on 'the continuing uncertainties with regard to the long-term health risks associated with fluoridation' and 'the possible adverse environmental effects'. By October 2014, the proposed fluoridation plan had been scrapped in its entirety due to the opposition. Public Health England (PHE) said that it still endorsed fluoridation but could not proceed without the backing of the local council.

What is the situation in the UK?

In the UK, around 10% of water supplies are fluoridated. Approximately 5.8 million people receive optimally fluoridated water, around 3.5 million of whom live in the West Midlands area. Other areas with fluoridated supplies are East Midlands, the North East, Cumbria, Cheshire, Lincolnshire, Humberside and Bedfordshire.

The Water Act 2003 handed the decision of whether to fluoridate water supplies to the strategic health authorities (SHAs) in England and the health boards in Scotland and Wales. Following the abolition of SHAs, the power was devolved back to the individual local authorities, which now have the final say with regard to fluoridation. The areas in most need of fluoridated water supplies are those with high tooth decay rates, including Merseyside and other parts of north-west England, Yorkshire, Scotland, Wales and Northern Ireland, plus some socially deprived communities in the south, such as inner London.

Who supports water fluoridation in the UK?

- British Medical Association
- Department of Health and Social Care
- BDA
- British Association for the Study of Community Dentistry (BASCD)
- British Fluoridation Society (BFS)
- World Health Organization (WHO)
- FDI World Dental Federation

What is the situation in other parts of the world?

According to the BFS, the USA has the most well-developed artificial fluoridation programme in the world, with approximately 171 million people receiving optimally fluoridated water. Other countries with fluoridated supplies are Canada, Brazil, Chile, Argentina, Peru, Guatemala, Guyana, the Irish Republic, Spain, Australia, New Zealand, Singapore, Malaysia, Brunei, South Korea, Vietnam, Papua New Guinea and Fiji.

What other products have fluoride added?

Several other methods of increasing fluoride intake have been used, including toothpaste, mouthwash, milk and salt. Salt fluoridation was first introduced in Switzerland in 1955 and is widespread in France, Switzerland, Germany, Spain, Austria, Hungary and the Czech Republic. This method has the advantage of not requiring a centralised piped water system and gives individuals control over its consumption.

However, it is not without its problems: dosage must take into account the other sources of fluoride in the area, to ensure that intake is not excessive. The production of fluoridated salt also requires specialist technology. Another consideration is the link between the consumption of sodium and hypertension, which would make this method of fluoride intake unsuitable for some individuals.

Fluoridated milk is also available and has been used widely (with parental permission) since 1993 in primary schools. Over 40,000 children in the UK, predominantly in the north-west of England, receive fluoridated milk at school, which has a concentration of 0.5mg of fluoride per carton. More recently, in 2016, Blackpool Council rolled out a plan to make fluoridated milk available for free to all primary school children as part of their breakfast clubs.

Another problem is monitoring and controlling fluoride administered in this manner; it is more difficult than with water because of the number of dairies involved. Fluoridated milk's dosage of fluoride also has to be adjusted, depending on whether the water supply is already naturally fluoridated or not. Additionally, a significant number of people do not drink milk for health or other reasons.

Mercury fillings

What are mercury fillings?

Amalgam fillings (the silver-coloured type) are the most common type of metal fillings and have been used for around 150 years. They are made of a combination of mercury (50%), silver (35%), tin (15%), copper and other metals. The major benefit of using amalgam is that it is economical, hard wearing and long lasting, and as such is ideal for using on molars.

Are there any risks associated with this type of filling?

There has always been a belief that mercury could not escape from the amalgam, but there is some evidence that mercury vapour does escape. Some countries have banned the use of mercury in fillings, among them

Sweden and Austria. Critics of mercury in fillings claim that the vapour can cause gum disease, kidney, liver and lung problems, Alzheimer's disease and multiple sclerosis. However, according to the British Dental Health Foundation, dental amalgam containing mercury is not poisonous when combined with the other metals present. It states that: 'Research into the safety of dental amalgam has been carried out for over 100 years. So far, no reputable controlled studies have found a connection between amalgam fillings and any medical problem.'

What are the alternatives?

The British Society for Mercury Free Dentistry recommends the removal of amalgam fillings and their replacement by composite fillings, but only if precautions are taken to ensure that mercury is not ingested or inhaled during removal. 'White' fillings – made of composite materials or polymers – can be used in place of silver fillings, but they are not as strong and so can often be unsuitable for the back teeth, which are subjected to greater stress than the front teeth.

'Was my treatment necessary?'

Because dentists are paid for the treatment they perform, the more treatment that a patient receives or the more complex the treatment is, the more money the dentist will be able to charge. The question has therefore been raised as to whether dentists provide unnecessary treatment to patients just to make more money. The *Guardian*, in an article entitled 'Do dentists put the bite on patients?', carried out an experiment (albeit a limited one) to test this: a reporter booked examinations at a number of surgeries in London, and the recommendations ranged from one filling and a trip to the hygienist (cost then £32.92) to two fillings and three replacement crowns (£915 then). Even bearing in mind that dentists have to use their professional judgement as to whether treatment is urgently required or could be delayed, the range of recommended treatment in this particular instance is staggering.

There have also been suggestions that some NHS dentists can purposely stretch out a course of treatment over more than two months to make more money. Under the current contract, if patients have to return to the dentist within two months to finish a course of treatment or have further treatment, the work is covered by one fee. However, if the treatment goes beyond two months, the dentist would be able to charge again. One Welshman carried out a series of attacks on his dental surgery, including leaving a hoax bomb on its front doorstep, because he thought he had been overcharged by his dentist!

In spite of these concerns and potential issues, it is clear that the great majority of dentists are scrupulous about providing only appropriate treatment in an appropriate timeframe to their patients.

Treatments of the future

Over the past 30 years, the way we have looked after our teeth has improved vastly. We visit the dentist more often, spend more money on dental hygiene products and invest in a wide range of cosmetic dentistry procedures to make our teeth more aesthetically pleasing. As with any other scientific discipline, new treatments and practices are introduced as time goes on and these further improve dental and oral care, and consequently dental health and hygiene. Some recent examples are introduced below.

3D printing

Three-dimensional printing has improved rapidly in the past decade and the use of this technology is increasingly being incorporated into medical treatments, although it is still in its infancy in the dental world. This type of printing has the potential to create items such as crowns, veneers or implants specifically for an individual patient, but could also be used to make bespoke specialist tools to be used in certain proce-dures. While this technology is not currently used as standard, in the long term it has the potential to be used by dentists in providing routine treatments on a daily basis.

Smart toothbrushes

As an extension of the various smart devices that we use within our homes, electric toothbrushes seem to be the next gadgets due for a smart overhaul. The idea behind this is that the toothbrush connects to your smartphone and monitors the duration, frequency and quality of brushing you carry out each day. This technology is extremely useful to provide guidance and tips to help an individual to brush more effectively and could be a vital weapon in helping to improve oral health, particularly in younger people.

It is worthwhile trying to keep up to date with advances such as these by reading relevant newspapers, journals and websites. This will enable you to have a good understanding of where the profession is heading and give you the best possible chance of shining at interview.

7 | Non-standard applications

Most students who consider pursuing dentistry at university will be classified as 'standard' applicants: these would usually be UK residents studying chemistry and biology at A level, Pre-U, International Baccalaureate, or at Higher Level in Scotland. However, if you do not fit the profile of a 'standard' applicant but wish to study dentistry, there are other possible entry options that can be pursued.

Those who have not studied science at A level

If you decide that you would like to study dentistry after starting on a combination of A levels that does not fit the subject requirements for entry to dental school, or if you meet certain contextual factors related to the school you studied at or the area you live in, you may be eligible to apply for the pre-dental course.

The application procedure, the interview and UCAT requirements are the same as for the five-year course at that particular university.

This course is offered at four faculties of dentistry: Bristol, Cardiff, Liverpool and Manchester (see Table 7 on page 122 for specific details). The course at Bristol is unique as it is aimed predominantly at students who have studied either biology or chemistry at A level but are unlikely to achieve the required grades due to contextual factors relating to the area they live in or the school they have previously studied at. At the other faculties the course is aimed predominantly at students who have only studied one science at A level and are predicted to secure AAA. The course covers elements of chemistry, biology and physics and lasts one academic year. Following successful completion, you automatically move on to the first year of the undergraduate dental course.

If your pre-dental application is unsuccessful, the best option is to take one-year science A level courses at a sixth-form or further education college. However, covering A level Biology and Chemistry from scratch in one year and getting the required A grades is a very tough challenge and should only be attempted by the most able students. You should discuss your particular circumstances with the staff at a number of colleges to select the course that will prepare you to achieve the A level subjects you need at the grades you require.

Table 7 Pre-dental course entry requirements – 2020/21

University	Standard offer	GCSE requirements	A level subject requirements	UCAT policy	Course code
Bristol	BBC	6/B in Science and 4/C in English Language and Mathematics	B in Biology or Chemistry	Required	A208
Cardiff	AAA	6/B in English Language; 6 GCSEs, including 7/A in the sciences	Nor more than one science from Biology, Chemistry or Physics	Required	A204
Liverpool	-	Five at 6/B or above to include Mathematics, English Language and Science	This course is designed for mature and non-traditional students who have taken a break from their studies for five or more years. It is not designed for A level students, school leavers or graduates	Not required	0AAW
Manchester	AAA	6/B in English Language and Mathematics and double award Science, or 4/C for separate sciences	3 arts/humanities subjects or 2 arts/humanities subjects plus 1 science	Required	A204

Overseas students

The competition for the few places available to overseas students is fierce and you would be wise to discuss your application informally with the dental school before submitting your UCAS application. Many dental schools give preference to students who do not have adequate provision for training in their own countries. You should contact the dental schools individually for advice.

According to the UCAS entrance statistics, students applying from outside the UK are much less successful than their UK counterparts in getting offers to study dentistry. For entry in 2018, 95 overseas students (EU and non-EU) gained a place to study dentistry at British universities, out of 1,295 applications. This represents a 7% chance of success compared with a 11% chance for UK students who applied in the same year. Further breakdown of these figures shows that in 2018, just 6% of applicants from the EU (excluding the UK) were successful, while non-EU international applicants had an 8% success rate.

At the time of writing, the government has promised that EU students starting their studies in September 2020 will be charged the same fees as domestic students for the duration of their course. However, EU students starting study in September 2021 who are not resident in the UK before the start of 2021, will no longer be eligible for home fee status.

Qualifications

Many overseas students are applying with qualifications that are not equivalent to A levels or other UK qualifications. These students cannot be considered unless they have done a course that leads to qualifications recognised as being equivalent to A levels, such as the International Baccalaureate (IB) or the Irish Leaving Certificate. The dental schools' websites will quote entrance requirements in terms of A levels, IB, Scottish Highers, the Irish Leaving Certificate and other equivalent qualifications. If you are studying for other qualifications, you will need to contact the dental schools directly to ask their advice; this will give you a definitive answer about whether what you have been studying is suitable.

If your qualifications are not recognised you will need to think about following a one-year A level programme (studying Biology, Chemistry and another subject) and applying while studying. Students will also need to demonstrate a certain proficiency in English.

English language requirements

All overseas students are expected to demonstrate that they have a certain standard of English before commencing a dentistry course. This is most commonly demonstrated by using the International English Language Testing System (IELTS), although there are other qualifications that may be considered. Again, if you are unsure about the suitability of any English language qualification you must check directly with the university.

Each university independently sets its own IELTS requirements, which are clearly shown alongside its admissions information. This can be found on the university websites and also on the UCAS website. The requirements vary, but on average, most universities require an overall score of between 6.0 and 7.0, with scores in each individual section of between 6.0 and 7.0. For example, for 2021 entry, Birmingham and Liverpool required a minimum overall score of 7.0 with a minimum of 7.0 in each component.

The application form

Students who are studying outside the UK are often at a disadvantage because they may not have access to advisers at their schools who are familiar with the requirements of a successful UCAS application. The two areas that tend to be weakest are the personal statement and the reference.

Students who are unfamiliar with UCAS applications often write unsuitable personal statements that concentrate too much on non-essential information (prizes, awards, responsibilities) and not enough on matters relevant to dentistry. It is important to explain why you wish to study dentistry in the UK rather than in your home country. Detailed advice on the personal statement can be found in Chapter 5 of this book. Similarly, your referee needs to be familiar with what the dental schools require in the reference; we have seen numerous references written by academic advisers outside of the UK that are more like character references and therefore contain mostly irrelevant details. The UCAS website is a wealth of information, in relation to both personal statement and reference writing; particularly useful are the short videos that outline the key points about writing both of these documents. It is well worth ensuring that your chosen referee is familiar with this information before proceeding.

Tips on writing the personal statement and reference can be found at www.ucas.com/undergraduate/applying-university/writing-personal-statement/how-write-personal-statement.

Work experience

Under normal circumstances, dental schools require applicants to have gained some relevant work experience, and often to have done some voluntary work as well, even if you are classed as a non-standard applicant. Work experience tells the selectors that the candidates are serious about becoming dentists and that they are familiar with what the profession demands. Voluntary work demonstrates that the applicant has the caring nature necessary to work with patients.

Gaining work experience can be difficult, but you should make every effort to do so. With the current challenges related to Covid-19, it has become increasingly difficult to secure work experience and some voluntary work placements. At the moment, universities are taking a flexible approach about what they are expecting students to have undertaken, however, they still require students to have taken steps to develop their understanding of the profession. If it has proved impossible for you to gain dental work experience and care-based voluntary work, it is vital that you explore as many other options as possible. This might include completing online courses, attending virtual seminars in relation to dentistry and speaking to a dentist on the telephone rather than shadowing them. In terms of voluntary work, there may be opportunities in the local community and online, even if they are not directly related to a care-based profession.

If you have struggled to find work experience, It is important that your reference explains why there is no mention of work experience in the application, and what you did to try to get that experience.

Interviews

Most dental schools require students to attend interviews. This is often difficult to arrange for students who are not based in the UK. It is worth contacting the schools before you apply to see whether they are likely to require you to travel to the UK to be interviewed. Given the current situation with Covid-19, it is expected that most interviews for the foreseeable future will be conducted via an online video-conferring platform such as Zoom or Microsoft Teams. This is likely to make it much easier for international students to be interviewed without extensive travelling.

Quotas

While there is currently no restriction on places for EU students, who will be currently considered alongside UK applicants, this is very likely to formally change during 2021 due to Brexit. For students outside of the EU, the UK government imposes quotas for how many non-UK/EU students can be accepted to study dentistry. In general, students from countries that do not have adequate training programmes for dentistry are likely to have an advantage. If you are serious about studying dentistry in the UK, then do not be put off by the statistics. It is worth bearing in mind that while almost all of the UK applicants will be suitably qualified to study dentistry and will be aware of the entrance require-ments (academic and other), a high proportion of overseas applicants will be rejected simply because they have not researched the require-ments properly. So, careful preparation will give you a good chance of being considered.

While there has been some fluctuation in the numbers of EU and non-EU students being accepted to study dentistry over the past 10 years, in reality, the figures have remained relatively constant. For non-EU applicants, this has been somewhere between 50 and 85 acceptances per year, with 75 being the most frequent number. For EU applicants, this has been between 5 and 20 acceptances per year, with 10 being most frequent.

Mature students

Every year, there are a number of entrants to dentistry who are mature students. In 2019, there were around 2,520 applications to study dentistry from students aged 21 or over; 215 of these were accepted. In general there are three types of mature student:

1. those who have always wanted to study dentistry but failed to get into dental school when they applied from school in the normal way
2. those who have studied a science-related degree and at some point decided that they wish to study dentistry
3. those who came to the idea later on in life, often having embarked on a totally unrelated degree or career.

The first two types of applicant will usually have completed a degree in an associated discipline, such as a science- or healthcare-related subject, and usually will have obtained a minimum classification of 2.i. They may not have got into a dental school when they applied as an A level student, or perhaps they wanted to pursue a science degree without ever really considering dentistry at the time. Mature students will have a greater chance of success if they have pursued an appropriate biomedical or healthcare-related first degree, such as:

- anatomy
- biomedical sciences
- biochemistry
- human biology
- medical science
- physiology.

This is intended as a guide only, and the suitability of any degree course should be checked directly with the university.

This type of applicant would then apply to either a standard five-year course or a four-year graduate-entry course following completion of their first degree. The four-year course is offered by Aberdeen, Central Lancashire (UCLan) and King's. These courses offer exemption from the first year of the course, so entry is into year two. Students who opt for this path can face an uphill struggle to make a successful application and so would need to have an excellent profile that demonstrates ongoing commitment to dentistry to maximise their chances of being accepted. Table 8 (opposite) gives details of these courses.

The third category of mature student is of equal interest to the dental school selectors and interviewers. Applications from people who have achieved success in other, non-science-related careers and who can bring a breadth of experience to the dental school and to the profession are welcomed. The main difficulty facing those who come late to the idea of studying dentistry is that they rarely have scientific backgrounds. There are two possible pathways that can be considered if you are in this position. Firstly, it would be possible to study science A levels and apply for a five-year course. Independent sixth-form colleges would be best placed to provide this pathway. Alternatively, it would be possible to apply to one of the six-year dental courses that incorporate a pre-dental year. Out of the four courses of this type that are available, Bristol, Cardiff and Manchester are open to those who have only a maximum of one science subject at A level.

Table 8 Entry requirements for graduate courses – 2020/21

University	Pre-degree requirements	Degree requirements	Interview	UCAT policy	Course code
Aberdeen	None	At least 2.i in a medical or health-related science degree. Applicants with a first degree in medicine will also be considered.	Yes	Required	A201
King's	None	At least 2.i in a biosciences subject or a 2.ii in a biosciences subject or health professional subject with a post-graduate degree (with at least a merit).	Yes	Required	A202
University of Central Lancashire (UCLan)	Three A levels at C or above, including two from Biology, Chemistry, Physics and Mathematics. GCSE Mathematics and English Language at 6/B.	2.i in a biomedical subject	Yes	Not required	A202

Case study: Andy Shaw, first-year dentistry student, University of Leeds

'I chose to study dentistry after completing some work experience in the field. Before work experience, I only had something scientific in mind and healthcare interested me. By exploring further I was able to decide that dentistry was for me. I learned about the role of healthcare professionals in more detail and had time to think about how my career should align with my values; I thought this was important to ensure an enjoyable career. Dentistry will also give me the opportunity to work in the hospital, close to the community in general practice, or both. I really look forward to making the most of the freedom of a career like dentistry, and this element was something that my future had to have. Finally, dentistry has a business element to it, which is a very exciting prospect and I will learn more about it later on.

'I carried out work experience in a few different settings before settling on dentistry. I shadowed surgeons in a local hospital, went on a GP placement, and completed two weeks of work experience in general dental practice. I learnt that the role of a dentist is not an easy job. I learnt there are many qualities needed for working with lots of different kinds of people on a daily basis, including empathy, professionalism, communication skills and veracity, to name a few. The patients trust the dentist to do their best, so all these skills are necessary to deliver the care that patients expect. More importantly, I learned that I should develop my weaker skills. Fortunately, I shadowed a dentist who enjoyed teaching me and emphasised the importance of ethics in dentistry.

'I studied Maths, Biology and Chemistry at A level. I achieved grades ABB in these subjects in the first sitting, but made the decision to resit Biology and Chemistry the following year and then achieved grades A and A*. I chose to study dentistry quite late on. Many dental and medical students seem to have decided on their career years before applying, so it can seem intimidating when you are competing against applicants who already know a lot about dentistry. My advice would be to gain as much insight as possible and make sure that you are as prepared as possible by using things such as the *BDJ* (*British Dental Journal*) to read around subjects, and an EPQ is always helpful when it comes to interviewing.

'Dentistry is very exciting so far. Despite no face-to-face teaching or clinical teaching due to Covid-19 restrictions, I have learnt a lot through online learning. I am enjoying learning about new subjects and looking forward to the challenges ahead. Currently, I particularly enjoy learning about the things I touched on when preparing for interview – it's important to know a little bit about everything when preparing for interview, so it's nice to finally learn things in detail. I anticipate later on in the course that patient contact and the practical aspects of dentistry will become very enjoyable. At the start of the course there was a lot of getting to know the resources and online learning system. It was difficult getting to grips with everything, such as the library system, but I know that it will be useful soon.

'Everybody is going through the same thing during the pandemic with a shift to online learning. For me it means I haven't been able to go into the dental school and do hands-on work, which I think I would really enjoy. More time at my desk rather than in lecture theatres or in clinic has given me the time to think about why I am doing this course and what I want to gain from university, both in terms of academic and extracurricular activities.

'In ten years I hope I will be a proficient dentist whose patients are happy to have me as a dentist. I don't know whether I will be working as a general dentist, but I enjoy the possibility of all specialities. I'm looking forward to finding out where my career leads.

'Lessons I've learnt from my own experiences of applying to dental schools are:

* Make sure that you use work experience to think about whether you can picture yourself doing the job forever. I could easily picture myself in the role of a dentist, but not in the other jobs I observed on work experience.
* Don't get complacent when it comes to A levels – the content may be relatively easy to understand, but getting an A or A* in exam season is much more difficult. Be proactive to give yourself the best chance.'

Case study: Hamza Khan, first year dentistry student, Plymouth University

'I wanted to enter a healthcare profession so I could use my interpersonal skills, but the artistry and intimacy of dentistry is what particularly interested me; the ability to carry out the care plan of a patient throughout their course of care and build rapport with them is of extreme importance to me.

'I carried out work experience at a family member's dental practice in the summer holidays prior to Year 13 and completed a six-week online course led by FutureLearn, which helped to show commitment in my dental school interviews. The course was insightful and I was able to gain an understanding of the qualities needed to be a dentist. Work experience was extremely beneficial as it highlighted the realities of the job and its demands. I also gained an insight into the variety of patients that one would meet, especially in a high needs area, or one of high social deprivation.

'At A level, I studied Biology, Chemistry and English Literature. I was due to sit my exams in 2020 after deferring them for a year because of extenuating circumstances, but the exams were cancelled because of Covid-19. On results day, I had not met the conditions of my offer to study at Plymouth because of the grades that had been calculated for me, despite receiving the required Centre Assessed Grades from my school. Following a subsequent government announcement, I was given a call a week prior to the start of the course asking if I was still interested as my grades were now AAA and dental schools were allowed to admit more students this cycle, so I was able to begin my studies rather than deferring them.

'In order to succeed on a dentistry course, you have to be very committed. It is not enough to learn by rote – you must have an appreciation of what you're learning. It is a great feeling knowing that what you are learning will be directly applicable to your career, compared to the generalised learning of A levels. The practical aspect, although limited due to Covid-19 at the moment, is obviously extremely enjoyable, and it helps to reinforce your learning. At the moment, the downsides are the long contact hours and the masses of content. Covid-19 means that much of our learning is currently online, but we still have two practical sessions a week, each lasting three hours, and a face-to-face life sciences session.

'In the future, I intend to be a qualified and successful dentist. I am keen to pursue specialisations in cosmetics, such as Botox and veneers, in a world that is increasingly focussed on the appearance of oneself.

'My tips for aspiring dentists would be to work hard, be honest with yourself and don't be disheartened or lose focus when knocked back.'

Studying abroad

One option for those who have been unsuccessful with their applications is to study dentistry at one of a number of dental schools abroad. These are five- and six-year courses that are taught in English. There are a number of well-known universities, such as Charles University in, Pague, Czech Republic University CEU Cardenal Herrera in Valencia, Spain; and Comenius University in Bratislava, Slovakia, that are found within the European Economic Area (EEA) and teach in English. There are also universities outside of the EEA that teach dental degrees in English. There is no central body like UCAS to apply through for these schools, so applications are completed individually for each dental school. The admissions process can differ for each university, but there may be the requirement to sit an entrance exam and/or attend an interview.

It is advised that students who are interested in studying abroad start their research up to 18 months in advance. This will allow enough time to thoroughly complete any application forms, sit any required tests or entrance exams (including language tests), obtain a visa (if required) and find funding. There are different guidelines to follow depending on where you wish to study and you will also need to research exactly what it is that you need to do. For example, if you wish to pursue a course within the EU and you are an EU national (which no longer includes UK students), you have a right to study in any other EU country. You also have the right to be charged the same level of fees that a home student in that country would pay. This means that the process is relatively straightforward, and there is no requirement to apply for a visa. If you are a British student, it is likely that, from January 2021, you will be charged a different rate of fees because of the UK's departure from the EU. However, this is worth checking with individual universities, as there are likely to be some differences between them in terms of fee policy.

If you wish to study outside the EU, however, there may be a require-ment to apply for a student visa. You may also find that you have to pay different fees compared to students who originate from the country. It is vital that you speak with the embassy or consulate of the country you wish to study in to check the steps that need to be followed.

There are some companies based in the UK that aim to help you gain entry to one of a number of these universities; however, it is best to approach the university directly to discuss entry as this is often a more straightforward and less expensive option. Applicants who are offered a place to study dentistry in Europe are not obliged to accept their place if they later choose to study in the UK. It is advisable for any committed prospective dentist who is applying to a UK dental school to have a back-up option to study dentistry in Europe, in the event that their appli-cation in the UK is unsuccessful.

When considering study abroad, you should remember that if you wish to come back to the UK to work as a dentist after graduation, you must first pass the Overseas Registration Exam (ORE) if you have studied outside of the European Economic Area (EEA). The ORE is designed to test knowledge and clinical skills based on the curriculum of UK dental schools. If you pass, you are then eligible to apply for full registration with the GDC, which will allow you to practise in the UK. Full details can be found at www.gdc-uk.org/professionals/ore. At the moment, if you studied in Switzerland or an EEA country (currently Austria, Belgium, Bulgaria, Croatia, Republic of Cyprus, Czech Republic, Denmark, Estonia, Finland, France, Germany, Greece, Hungary, Iceland, Ireland, Italy, Latvia, Liechtenstein, Lithuania, Luxembourg, Malta, The Netherlands, Norway, Poland, Portugal, Romania, Slovakia, Slovenia, Spain and Sweden) your qualification can allow you to register with the GDC as long as the course is approved by the regulator in whichever country you are studying in. The UK national agency for international qualifications and skills (UK ENIC, www.enic.org.uk) can advise on regulations and outline the steps you may need to take before finding employment as a dentist in this country.

As has been previously mentioned, the June 2016 referendum on the UK's relationship with Europe has somewhat confused the situation in terms of studying in the EEA. It is likely that as the nature of the relationship between the UK and EU continues to evolve post-January 2021, there will be changes to the rules in relation to eligibility to return to practise dentistry in the UK after graduation.

Case study: Sumandeep Kailey, fifth year dentistry

'I grew up surrounded by dentists and dental nurses, and it was always a field I have felt very comfortable in and understood well. The pros: being able to help my local community in a hands-on manner while getting to know its members on a personal level; te cons: grumpy and potentially rude patients combined with long working hours. I feel dentistry is a career that allows you to still maintain some element of a social life outside of your job, with its flexible working hours, and also one in which I will be able to carry out precise manual work, which I always enjoyed through school subjects such as design technology and art.

'Before completing my application, I carried out work experience at a local general dental practice where I was able to experience both NHS and private practice; a welcome contrast, as it showed how different dentistry can be, though maintaining the same basics of knowledge. I also was able to sit in on some periodontal surgery, which was absolutely fascinating once you're able to get over the shock of physically seeing the bone of the maxilla in real life!

'Through my work experience, I learnt that dentistry relies heavily on teamwork. The working day is made more efficient, and generally more fun, if you get along with your colleagues and peers and are able to work well together even in tricky situations where people may not see eye to eye. I also learnt that dentistry is not as glamorous as Instagram dentists may suggest it to be – I saw a man vomit into the dentist's hand as he took an impression for a denture.

'At A level I studied Geography, Biology, Chemistry and English Literature, and secured grades A*ABB in these subjects respectively. I initially had conditional offers to study dentistry from Leeds and Plymouth, who both required AAA. I accepted Leeds as my firm choice and Plymouth as my insurance choice. However, when results day rolled around, I failed to notice that the "terms of my offer had changed" due to my B grade in chemistry. Thankfully, both Leeds and Plymouth had liked me at interview, and I was given an offer to study at Leeds the following year, with my missed grade leaving me on the waiting list for an offer if anyone for that

---

year was to drop out; and Plymouth accepted me to start that year. I was willing to wait a year to go to Leeds as it was my first choice, but just when I had planned a gap year, I got a phone call from Leeds about five days before the start of term, offering me a place for that year. The rest is history!

'So far, studying dentistry has been a challenging experience all in all. There are days I am absolutely overjoyed, such as when I have carried out complex treatment on a patient with a complex medical history really well and I feel like a real dentist! However, naturally, as with anything, it has its down days and you wish you had chosen a degree with fewer bodily fluids involved. I feel it is a degree that really requires dedication and determination to get through – five years is a long time to study a subject you are "unsure" about.

'Personally, my favourite part of the course is the patient interaction – being able to connect with so many people from so many backgrounds with different stories and knowledge to share is endless fun; and if you're helping them out and making their lives a little easier with your dental knowledge and skill then that can't be a bad thing! I also love the real-world application of the clinical knowledge we learn – smoking cessation advice will always win you loads of friends, I promise. I have always struggled with the more academic histology involved in the course. The first two years are packed full of more science-based material and biochemistry that is essential in understanding why we then carry out the dentistry we do. However, it is a necessary evil and one that is vital, particularly if you choose to go down the research route.

'As dentistry is highly based on patient contact, our clinical procedures during the Covid-19 pandemic are greatly limited, with no aerosol generating procedures permitted in our clinics in Leeds until we are fitted with adequate PPE. This means we are mainly doing prosthetic work and extractions for now, which is not ideal in terms of building experience pre-graduation, but necessary in these unprecedented times. Additionally, the interviews we usually take part in in early November have been cancelled, and instead we are purely doing situational judgement tests in order to determine our national ranking before our foundation year training.

'At the moment, I am taking my fifth year of study day by day, and I am only looking forward to graduation! But in ten years' time, I would hope to be slightly more adept in carrying out a root canal treatment and perhaps be delving more into the world of public health and policy. I would love to work in the Department of Health and Social Care and start implementing and suggesting policies to support our NHS.

'Though it is unfashionably clichéd, my advice to prospective dentistry students would be never give up. I remember thinking that it was so impossible and unachievable to get where I am now, especially when I was getting C grades in my A level mocks, and walking home in the rain, with my tummy grumbling, and UCAT/ BMAT revision waiting for me when I got home; but you have got to be focussed and determined and have your eyes set on the goal. It may feel like forever when you're slogging through those past papers, but it will be worth it! That being said, balance is key; it is so important to look after your mental health, even while applying to uni. Dentistry will always be there, but the mind is fragile and deserves more love than any form of academia.'

Students with disabilities and special educational needs

Students with disabilities and special educational needs are welcome to apply to study dentistry. The vast majority of universities will have an equality and diversity adviser or team (or equivalent) that is employed to provide guidance and support to students with specific needs.

It is absolutely vital that any specific learning difficulty or disability be disclosed in the appropriate section of your UCAS application. It is crucial that no details be hidden from the university at this point. If the university knows about your needs from the start, it will be better placed to provide the appropriate support from the beginning of your course. It is also important to remember that your application will not be discriminated against based on the information you provide in it.

It must be remembered, however, that dentistry makes very specific physical demands on individuals. As a result, any physical disability that may interfere with the ability to meet these demands may make dentistry an unsuitable course. The GDC recommends that a student should only be accepted onto a course if he or she is able to carry out all of the tasks normally done by dentists. It also requires applicants to satisfy the 'fitness to practise' criteria. If you are unsure about how your disability will affect you in these areas, then it is worth contacting the universities so that you can be assessed individually.

It is also worth contacting the team at each university where you wish to study in advance of applying to discuss the facilities and mechanisms it would be able to put in place to support you during your studies. This is a vital task and so should form part of your research and fact-finding about a particular university.

8 | What do I do on results day?

You will probably have been worrying about results day for a number of weeks by the time it eventually rolls around. Although it can be a very emotional day for some, it is important to be thoroughly prepared for whatever situation may arise on the day.

Your A level results will usually arrive at your school on the third Thursday in August, with the dental schools receiving them sometime before this. Scottish Higher results are traditionally released a week earlier than A level results. It is vital that you are present in person on the day so that you can collect your results; don't wait for your school to post them, and try to avoid getting them by phone or email as this can sometimes lead to you being given incorrect information. Collecting your results at school will put you in the best position to act as quickly as possible if you haven't managed to secure your place. Prior to results day, check what time your school opens and what time results are available; the sooner you get to your school and pick them up, the sooner you could be on the phone to university admissions teams. In addition to this, you will be able to find out whether you have been accepted or rejected by your chosen universities prior to going into your school or college by logging on to UCAS Track, so have your login details to hand.

If things go wrong during the exams

If something happens when you are preparing for or actually taking the exams that prevents you from doing your best, you must notify your school/college, the exam board and the dental schools that have made you offers. This notification will come best from your head teacher and should include your UCAS number and date of birth. Send it off at once; it is no good waiting for disappointing results and then telling everyone that you felt ghastly at the time but said nothing. Exam boards can give you special consideration if the appropriate forms are sent to them by the school, along with supporting evidence. An increasing number of dental schools now only accept mitigating circumstances if they were reported to the exam board at the time of the examination.

Your extenuating circumstances must be significant. A 'slight sniffle' won't do! If you really are sufficiently ill to be unable to prepare for the exams or to perform effectively during them, you must consult your GP and obtain a letter describing your condition.

The other main cause of underperformance is distressing events at home. If a member of your immediate family is very seriously ill, or if you have some form of significant domestic upheaval, you should explain this to your head teacher and ask him or her to write to the examiners and dental schools.

With luck, the exam board will give you the benefit of the doubt if your marks fall on a grade boundary. Equally, you can hope that the dental school will allow you to slip one grade below the conditional offer, although this is rare now that there are so many applicants chasing a small number of places. If things work out badly, then the fact that you declared extenuating circumstances should ensure that you are treated sympathetically if you decide to reapply through UCAS.

The dental school admissions departments are well organised and efficient, but they are staffed by human beings. If there were extenuating circumstances that could have affected your exam performance and that were brought to their notice in June, it is a good idea to ask them to review the relevant letters shortly before the exam results are published.

If you hold an offer and get the grades

If you previously received a conditional offer and your grades equal or exceed that offer, congratulations! You can relax and wait for your chosen dental school to send you joining instructions. One word of warning: you cannot assume that grades of A*AB satisfy an AAA offer. This is especially true if the B grade is in biology or chemistry. You should call your chosen university as soon as possible to check if you have met your offer.

If you hold no offer

There are a number of students who will approach results day without having received an offer from a dental school. There are a small number of dentistry places each year allocated through Clearing, although these are unlikely to be formally advertised on the UCAS website. It is extremely unlikely that a student will secure a place on a dentistry course in this way, but it is certainly not impossible, especially if your grades include at least one A* in a science subject. If you find yourself in this position, telephone all of the dental schools as soon as possible on results day to explain your situation. Although most are likely to say no, some universities have been known to invite students for interview on or shortly after results day and then subsequently make an offer. Remember the chances of this happening are slim, and most students will end up using Clearing to secure a place on an alternative course.

If you hold three A/A* grades but were rejected when you applied through UCAS (i.e. you did not get an offer), you need to let the dental schools know that you are out there, and discuss options for how you may secure a place in the future. The best way to do this is by phone or email, as these are the quickest ways of contacting the dental schools directly. It is always best to try to establish a good working relationship with admissions teams at the universities you are interested in, as they will be more likely to give you advice and help you in the future.

In this situation, the main option you have is to reapply through UCAS in the next admissions cycle. Although you will already have the grades for entry in this situation, it is important to understand that there are a number of other elements of your application that you'll need to work on to maximise your chances of securing a place. Things to consider are listed below.

- Your personal statement: revisit it and cast a critical eye over it. This is also an opportunity to add any work placements or other positive experiences that you have had since your last application.
- Your UCAT/BMAT score: you will need to resit any pre-admissions tests for each admissions cycle. This will give you a chance to complete further practice questions and learn from your experience of sitting it first time around. It may also be a good idea to attend one of the UCAT/BMAT preparation courses that are available.
- Your work experience and voluntary work: any opportunity to add further work experience to your profile will always be a good idea. Whether it is dentistry-related or just general voluntary work, it will have a positive impact.

What is UCAS Extra?

UCAS Extra is a service that allows students to apply to additional courses if they have been rejected by all their choices or declined all of their offers. This option is open between February and July and is a normal part of the whole application process. If at any time in the cycle you are eligible for UCAS Extra, it will show up when you log in to Track.

Since UCAS Extra started, there have not been any dentistry places advertised, and it is unlikely that this will change in the future due to the continued high levels of demand for places. However, it is not impossible – places for equally competitive courses, such as medicine and veterinary medicine, have been advertised in recent years, so it is certainly worth keeping an eye on. If you have been rejected from your first-choice courses, Extra provides an excellent opportunity to apply for other alternative courses without having to go through Clearing.

If you wish to use this facility, you must first search through the available courses on the UCAS website to find one that you are interested in and then call the university to check that it will consider you. If it gives you a positive response, then you can add the details on Track; the university will then contact you in the usual way when it has considered your application. If you do opt to use Extra, you will only be able to apply for one course at a time; you will not be able to add multiple courses all at once.

Is UCAS Adjustment of any use to me?

In effect, the UCAS Adjustment option is designed to be a 'trading up' system for applicants who pass their exams with better results than expected. However, you can only enter Adjustment if your results have met and exceeded the conditions of your conditional firm choice. A student must have held a conditional firm choice on their application to be eligible, and so if you have had no offers it is not something you can use.

If you hold an offer but miss the grades

If you have only narrowly missed the required grades, it is important that you contact the dental admissions team as soon as possible. As mentioned previously, you will probably know what their decision is at this point, thanks to the UCAS website. If you have been rejected, it is vital that you keep a level head and do not panic; you must stay calm throughout. If you have not been rejected outright or are unsure of their decision, you must contact the admissions team by telephone – so ensure that in the run-up to results day you have gathered together the contact numbers of the universities you have accepted as your firm and insurance choices.

In some cases, dental schools will allow applicants who hold a conditional offer to slip a grade (particularly if they came across well at the interview stage and it was their first-choice university) rather than offering the place to somebody else. However, be warned – this is by no means guaranteed, and most of the time dropping a grade will result in outright rejection, although the chances of being accepted in this position have improved in recent years.

When speaking to the universities, they are likely to give you a simple yes or no answer or tell you that you are still being considered. It is unlikely that crying, begging or pleading your case to the person on the phone will make any difference to the overall decision. If they tell you that you have been rejected, there are some questions you should ask.

- Would they consider your application if you applied next year (i.e. do they accept resit students)?

- What would the likely grade requirements be?
- Would they need to interview you again?
- Would they require you to resit the UCAT/BMAT? (Although the general policy is that it should be retaken, some universities have been known to waive this requirement.)

If they have given you a positive response about reapplying, seek to get it confirmed in writing, as this will give you hard evidence of their intention to consider your application again. It is probably easiest for them to confirm this by email, so you will first need to send them an email to enquire. If you are told by the universities you held offers with that they will not consider your application in the next cycle, you should call other dental schools to see if they would consider you. Unfortunately, the number of dental schools that will consider applications from retake students who have not held a conditional firm offer with them has becoming increasingly limited (see Table 3 in Chapter 3).

If you have had a positive response from one or more dental schools about reapplying, you would then need to consider retaking your A levels and applying again later in the year (see below). The alternative is to use the Clearing system to obtain a place on a degree course related to the biological/biomedical sciences and then apply to the dental course after you graduate and hope to be offered a place.

Retaking A levels

If you narrowly miss the required grades in your A levels after two years of study, you may wish to take the opportunity to retake any subject in which you underperformed to try to boost your grade. Remember that it is extremely difficult to make a successful application as a retake student, so improving your grades may not be enough to get you into dentistry. Before you embark on any retake courses, you need to carry out thorough research into which universities would consider you as a retake student. This information changes every year, so the only way to make sure that you have the most up-to-date information is to contact the university directly and explain your situation.

If you held offers with dental schools in the previous year and only narrowly missed your grades, you are more likely to be considered again the following year. For example, Cardiff University will defer the conditional place of an applicant who has missed their grades to the following year, providing they are able to obtain the grades in a subsequent sitting.

Case study: Avani Gill, fifth-year dentistry student, University of Sheffield

'I chose to study dentistry because it seemed like the perfect balance between science and hands-on practical work in a creative way, which made the prospect of dentistry very fun for me.

'When applying to study dentistry, I undertook work experience at a general dental practice (GDP) – with my actual dentist! I wasn't aware of any other places at the time that would take me because of insurance reasons. Looking back, what you could actually see and understand when observing was quite limited. I learnt more about the ins and outs of dental practice and regulations. The GDP I was shadowing gave me ideas on where to find further information about the regulatory side of things, such as CQC documentation, GDC Standards and protocols. I also had the opportunity to speak to an orthodontist as well as a newly qualified GDP. Being able to talk to these people and gain their insights was an invaluable part of my application process.

'I studied History, Biology and Chemistry at A level and achieved grades A*AA. I didn't get into dentistry on my first try. I applied and received an offer from Queen's Belfast, but on results day I had the ultimate heartbreak of not getting my grades and having to sit down and really think about what I wanted to do from there. Ultimately my desire to get into dentistry was greater than to just go to university for anything, so taking a year out to resit was the best option for me. I have no regrets – yes, I wasn't at uni when all my friends were, but I waited and got what I wanted in the end. I ended up taking two years out as I resat and achieved my grades but didn't apply that year. I applied the following year knowing I had my grades under my belt; this gave me the opportunity to work and travel. I even worked as a dental nurse for five months in my gap year, which turned out to be a huge help! Any clinical skills sessions we had in my first two years of uni flew by, and I was really confident because I knew the instruments, procedures, dental materials and protocols. Even just speaking with patients, I was very confident compared to my peers.

'Studying dentistry isn't all fun and games! I struggled with my first year a lot as it was heavily science-based/theory recall. Bear in mind it had been over a year since I had revised for anything! Nonetheless, I got through and from second year onwards, when we got more clinical experience and everything was more dental centred, I loved it!

'I can definitely say as a dental student you get your money's worth of teaching/face-to-face sessions. Having a busy timetable keeps you occupied, and when you become more confident in your skills, it's the best feeling. You quickly realise that it's not just academics you need to get you through; you need to be confident in yourself and your communication skills to do well, and this isn't something you are told when applying.

'I love the hands-on experience you get during your degree – naturally, most of your degree is practise practise practise! Alongside this, you really get to know your patients, build relationships and see things through. It's not like medicine, where you can see multiple patients a day but sometimes never see any of them again. With dentistry comes the chance to see how you can impact your patient's oral health, and it's really fulfilling when you see how you can motivate your patients.

'One aspect of dentistry that you cannot escape is evidence-based dentistry. It is an amazing concept, but one I just can't get my head round at times, so it's an aspect I enjoy less. For anything we do, such as which material we use for a filling or a technique we use to place a crown, there is evidence, and you have to understand the evidence and research it to really give your patients the best care. This is all fine and great, but not all evidence is good. You have to learn how to spot the good from the bad and really hone your research skills during your degree. It can be very confusing at times, and can be very cumbersome to do!

'The pandemic has really affected our clinical experience. Sheffield Dental School has been amazing in terms of organising everything and we have been lucky enough to be back in clinic in some capacity since August, but where we used to do procedures such as fillings, crown preps, periodontics work every day, we now have one session a week to do these things. It's been a real shame to not be able to practise normally and the patient experience isn't the same. Wearing full PPE isn't great, as you can't talk to patients in the same way, and having that barrier makes everything very formal. Some procedures are also on hold at our dental hospital – no root canals are taking place or dentures being made. This is a major issue as we are here to look after teeth, but in many scenarios now where patients attend in pain, instead of offering to save a tooth the only option for them at times is an extraction. This feels so counterintuitive and almost the opposite of what we learn!

'In ten years' time, I am hoping I will have completed training for a speciality post – my interests are mainly in restorative work and fixed prosthodontics at the moment, but who knows what the future holds!

'My tips for aspiring dentists would be:
- Don't forget to enjoy your degree! I feel that sometimes you can really get bogged down by not knowing as much as someone else on your course, or getting stressed out about things really easily. It's important to keep on top of things, but it's also important to really enjoy what you do because in dentistry it's very specialised and it's not easy to move careers when you do something like this. It's also much easier to excel in something you enjoy!
- Use your peers in the years above you for guidance and support! Dental students have a little community, so make friends, use your older peers for guidance and support – the older peers have been through everything you will have to go through at some point!'

Reapplying to dental school

Most dental schools do not consider retake candidates (see Table 3 in Chapter 3), so the whole business of applying again needs careful thought and research, hard work and a bit of luck.

When reapplying, the choice of dental schools open to you will be much narrower than the first time round. Most do not consider retake students at all; others will only consider you if there are extenuating circumstances that affected your academic performance; and some will only consider you if you previously applied to study with them and were made an offer. In addition, those dental schools who will consider retake applicants may have conditions regarding your attainment at A level in your first sitting. It is vital that you check the advice given by each dental school before you think about applying to it, as their position on retake students is always changing.

If you feel that there are extenuating circumstances that have prevented you from reaching your target grades, you must try to get evidence to support this in advance of results day. For example, if you have had a medical condition that has affected your performance, a letter from your doctor will be sufficient. Some examples of acceptable reasons for underachieving are:

- your own illness
- the death or serious illness of a very close relative
- serious domestic upheaval, such as parental divorce.

The following are examples of excuses that would not be regarded by admissions tutors as extenuating circumstances.

- 'I had so many exams to revise for that I didn't have time to do everything.'
- 'I have three young brothers and the noise they make stops me from revising.'
- 'I went skiing at Easter, and was unable to revise properly because it was too cold in the evenings for me to work.'
- 'I lost all of my notes a week before the exam and so couldn't revise.'
- 'We moved house a month before the exams, which disrupted my revision schedule.'

These are just guidelines, and the only safe method of finding out whether a dental school will consider your application is to call or write and ask. It is often worth writing an email or letter so that you have firm details of what has been discussed to refer back to at a later point if necessary. An example is provided below, although a telephone discussion could also take this form. Don't follow it word for word, and do take the time to write to all dental schools before you make your final choice. The format of your email should be:

- an opening paragraph
- your exam results: set them out clearly and with no omissions
- any extenuating circumstances (a brief statement)
- your retake plan, including the timescale
- a request for help and advice
- a closing paragraph.

Make sure that your letter is brief, clear and well presented. If you have had any previous contact with the admissions staff you will be able to write 'Dear Dr Smith' and 'Yours sincerely'. Even if you go to this trouble, the pressure on dental schools in the autumn is such that you may receive no more than a standard reply to the effect that, if you reapply, your application will be considered. Apart from the care needed in making the choice of dental school, the rest of the application procedure is as described in the first part of this guide.

Remember that if you are reapplying to universities that use the UCAT/ BMAT, then in all probability you will also have to resit the test, regardless of how you did in the previous year. Unfortunately, it is always your most recent score that counts, not your highest.

The same advice applies if you are reapplying with qualifications other than A levels. If you did not get a place but now have the grades required, then you will probably be able to reapply, but make sure you talk to the dental schools first. If you have not got the grades, then you need to look at what routes are available. For example, if you do not resit the IB, you will need to look at A levels or Foundation programmes in order to reach the requisite entry requirements for a dentistry course. If you have taken Scottish Highers, depending on the subject, you will be able to retake again in a new academic year. Either way, you must make sure that you gain the necessary qualifications in the next sitting. Even though this will allow entry to only a handful of dental schools, you should still make contact and speak to the admissions tutors at those dental schools that consider retakes.

Dear Miss Nash

Last year's UCAS No. 08-123456-7

I am currently in the process of completing my UCAS application and am particularly interested in applying to your university to study dentistry. I applied to you last year and received an offer of AAB but missed the grades/was rejected after interview/was rejected without an interview. However, I am very impressed by the university and the structure of the course and as such would like to apply again. I have just received my A level results, which were Biology A, Chemistry B, Psychology B.

During my final year of A levels, I had significant health problems that prevented me from achieving the grades I am capable of. I am now embarking on retaking each of my subjects in order to improve my grades. Now that I am back to full health, I have no doubt that I can achieve A grades in each subject.

Could you please advise me as to whether you would consider my application, given the circumstances I have outlined above. I am very keen not to waste a slot on my UCAS application (or your time) by applying to you if you will reject me purely because I am retaking.

I am very keen to study here, and would be extremely grateful for any advice that you can give me.

Yours sincerely

Diana Littlewood

---

9 | Fees and funding

Whether undertaking an undergraduate or postgraduate course, the cost of studying is considerable. This has been exacerbated in recent years by rises in living costs and the large increases in university tuition fees following the publication of the Browne review in 2010. In 2020, the UK Parliament's House of Commons Library released student loan statistics revealing that, on average, students graduating in 2019 had a debt of £40,000. However, these figures were based on an average of all students, rather than focusing on dental students. If we take into account the course length, then an English student at an English dental school in London could leave university with a significantly higher level of debt if the full amount of tuition fee and maintenance loan is received and there is no financial support from other sources. Bear in mind, however, that this overall cost to students will fluctuate depending on a number of factors. Some of these are listed below.

- Geographical location: obviously studying in London is going to be more expensive than studying in Birmingham.
- Area of permanent residence: there are differences in fees payable and help available depending on where you are from.
- Parental help: contributions from parents may significantly help meet the cost of living.
- Availability of scholarships: does the university offer scholarships for exceptional students?
- Finding a job: although it has the potential to interfere with your studies, working during your time at university will help to reduce the overall burden of debt.

When considering levels of student debt, it is easy to become disheartened and think that university study is not for you. What all students must remember is that tuition fees do not have to be paid up front; in fact, most students receive student loans to cover this cost. In addition, the loans do not start to be paid back until you are earning over a certain amount. The full details of this will be discussed later in the chapter.

Regardless of how much debt you incur, or how you fund your way through university, hopefully these figures will help you to realise that undertaking a course such as dentistry should only be done after seriously considering the overall cost and carefully examining your ability to be fully committed to your study for the full five years.

To find out what the fees are and what funding is available for dentistry courses, you should explore each of the universities' websites and/or talk to their financial departments, because fees and funding procedures vary from university to university. However, due to the high quality of education provided by dental schools, it is extremely likely that all of these courses will charge the maximum amount permitted.

It is vital to ensure that you carefully plan your finances in advance so that you are prepared to cover the cost of tuition fees, living expenses, books and other necessary equipment. Needless to say, living costs in big cities such as London will be much higher than in other parts of the country.

Fees

UK

Students who are UK nationals pay lower tuition fees than both EU and non-EU international students. For 2021 entry, universities will continue to charge up to £9,250 per year for tuition fees; it is expected that this figure will continue to rise in the future in line with inflation. The rise in fees is part of the government's new Teaching Excellence Framework (TEF), which assesses universities and colleges on the quality of their teaching. The institutions with a TEF award are able to charge £9,250, whereas those without a TEF award are only able to charge £9,000. Tuition fee loans have also increased to cover the higher fees.

There are a number of differences between the systems in England, Scotland, Wales and Northern Ireland, which can result in massive differences between the fees that are ultimately paid by students. From September 2018, the rules are as follows, although they may be subject to change in the future.

- English students are liable for the full fees being charged regardless of where they study within the UK, although for Welsh universities, the maximum amount being charged is still £9,000.
- Students living in Scotland who wish to study full time at a Scottish university are not required to pay tuition fees as long as eligibility criteria are met. Scottish students who wish to study at a university in England or Northern Ireland are required to pay fees of up to £9,250 per academic year. If studying in Wales they will pay £9,000 per year.
- For students residing in Wales, up to £9,250 per academic year will be payable if studying at an English, Scottish or Northern Irish university. Welsh students wanting to study in Wales have their fees subsidised by the Welsh Assembly and so are only required to pay up to £9,000 per year.
- Students living in Northern Ireland who wish to study in Northern Ireland will pay up to £4,395 per academic year. Northern Irish students who wish to study elsewhere in the UK are required to pay

up to £9,250 per academic year for studying in England or Scotland and £9,000 for studying in Wales.

EU students

In June 2020, the Universities Minister for England, Michelle Donelan, announced that, from August 2021, EU, other EEA and Swiss nationals will no longer qualify for home fee status for degree level study, and will no longer be able to access financial support from Student Finance England. Instead, universities will set their own fees for EU students. Many of these are yet to be finalised, but they are likely to be in line with fees for non-EU international students. The respective governments in Northern Ireland, Wales and Scotland later confirmed that the same changes to EU student fees as in England would be applied from 2021.

Non-EU international students

For international students from outside the UK and EU, the costs of studying in the UK are significantly greater and can often be prohibitive. For example, at the University of Birmingham the tuition fees for students starting in the academic year 2020–21 will be £23,400 per annum for year 1, rising to £42,000 per annum for years 2 to 5. At King's College London, international students will pay £45,600 per annum. While there is some variation in cost between universities, these fees are broadly representative of the whole of the UK.

Table 9 Annual tuition fees by region for courses starting in 2021

Student's home region	Studying in England	Studying in Scotland	Studying in Wales	Studying in Northern Ireland
England	Up to £9,250	Up to £9,250	Up to £9,000	Up to £9,250
Scotland	Up to £9,250	No fee	Up to £9,000	Up to £9,250
Wales	Up to £9,250	Up to £9,250	Up to £9,000	Up to £9,250
Northern Ireland	Up to £9,250	Up to £9,250	Up to £9,000	Up to £4,395
EU and other international	Variable	Variable	Variable	Variable

Source: www.ucas.com/ucas/undergraduate/finance-and-support/
undergraduate-tuition-fees-and-student-loans.
We acknowledge UCAS' contribution of this information.

Financial help

There are a number of sources of financial help that are potentially available for full-time students from both the UK and EU to help cover the cost of university study. The main ones are student loans and bursaries, which are all allocated according to individual and family circumstances. It is important to apply as soon as possible through the Student Finance online service in order to prevent delay in receiving this assistance. There are different Student Finance sites to use depending on which country you are a permanent resident of. These sites contain detailed information on the help that is available and how to apply for it:

- **England:** Student Finance – www.gov.uk/studentfinance
- **Scotland:** Student Awards Agency for Scotland (SAAS) – www.saas.gov.uk
- **Wales:** Student Finance Wales – www.studentfinancewales.co.uk
- **Northern Ireland:** Student Finance Northern Ireland – www.studentfinanceni.co.uk

For the most recent figures, please check the relevant Student Finance websites regularly.

Student loans

The most common way for students to finance their studies is by taking out a student loan. If you are an eligible, full-time student, you can take out two types of loan: a loan for tuition fees and a maintenance loan to meet living costs. The tuition fees loan does not depend on your household income and is paid straight to the university to cover the full cost. You can borrow all or part of the amount required to cover your fees.

The amount of maintenance loan you are entitled to depends on several factors, including household income, where you live while you're studying and what year of study you are in (see Table 10).

If you're living away from home, the maximum maintenance loan for English students is £9,203 for the academic year 2020–21, although if you're studying in London it's £12,010. The maximum available is less if you're living with your parents during term time. The costs vary depending on which part of the UK you normally live in and, in most cases, your household income. The details are shown in Table 10 opposite.

It is vital to remember when considering student loans that both the tuition fee and living expenses loans are not like loans you would get from a bank as you only start paying it back when you have a job that pays over a certain amount. Currently these thresholds are £26,575 per annum (before deductions) for English and Welsh students and £19,390 for Scottish and Northern Irish students. The repayments are then taken directly from your pay packet by your employer.

Table 10 Maximum maintenance loan available (2020–21)

Living arrangements during term time	Maximum maintenance loan available in England	Maximum maintenance loan available in Scotland	Maximum maintenance loan available in Wales	Maximum maintenance loan available in Northern Ireland
Living at home	£7,747	£7,750	£8,335	£5,338
Living away from home and studying outside London	£9,203	£7,750	£9,810	£6,428
Living away from home and studying in London	£12,010	£7,750	£12,260	£8,368

Source: www.gov.uk/student-finance/new-fulltime-students
Contains public sector information licensed under the Open Government Licence v3.0.

Student grants

Historically, the maintenance grant was available to help students with accommodation and other living costs and did not have to be repaid. However, in September 2016, the maintenance grant system was abolished for English students, and as a result, any funding received is now in the form of a loan. Means-tested grants for Scottish, Northern Irish and Welsh students still exist, although this situation may change in the future. The details of grants available are listed below for each country:

England

Most grants have been abolished. Some support may be available to certain students, for example, students with children and students with a disability.

Scotland

Students under the age of 25 may be entitled to the Young Students Bursary (YSB), which is the equivalent of a grant. Currently, if your household income is under £21,000, you receive a maximum of £2,000. This amount then tapers to zero if you have a household income of £34,000 or over per annum. Support may also be available to certain students, for example, lone parents and students with a disability.

Wales

The Welsh Government Learning Grant (WGLG) is a grant available depending on household income. Currently, if household income is less than £18,370 per annum, the maximum amount of £8,100 is payable if you're living away from home. This reduces on a sliding scale to a minimum of £1,000 if income exceeds £59,200 per annum. Up to £6,885 is available for those who live at home while studying, while £10,214 is available to those students studying in London.

Additionally, a Special Support Grant (SSG) is available for certain individuals depending on circumstances. For example, this can be paid if you are a single parent, have a disability or are in receipt of certain benefits. For the academic year 2020–21, the maximums are £12,260 for those studying in London, £9,810 for those studying outside of London and £8,335 for those living at home while studying.

Northern Ireland

Special Support Grants or Maintenance Grants are available in part if household income is less than £41,065. The full grant of £3,475 is awarded if household income is £19,203 or less, and this tapers to zero up to an income of £41,065. Additional support is available to certain students, for example, lone parents and students with a disability.

In all countries where the grant is still available, if your application for a maintenance grant is successful, the value of this will be deducted from your maintenance loan.

NHS bursaries

NHS bursaries are available for students studying their fifth year of dentistry in England, Wales and Northern Ireland, and from the second year onwards for students studying in Scotland. To be eligible for such a bursary, a student must qualify as a home student and be on a 'pre-registration health professional training course'. During the first four years of study, dental students are entitled to apply for tuition fee and maintenance loans from Student Finance. From year five onwards, dental students are eligible to apply for a means-tested NHS bursary alongside a reduced student loan to cover maintenance costs. In addition, fees in year five are paid in full by the NHS Student Bursary scheme, though the funding provision varies between England, Wales, Scotland and Northern Ireland. For more information, visit the NHS Health Careers website (www.healthcareers.nhs.uk/career-planning/study-and-training/considering-or-university/financial-support-university).

Scholarships

Certain universities make scholarships available, and these can be a valuable source of income throughout a course. There are some general scholarships as well as ones available only to dentistry students. Details can be obtained from the individual universities, but websites such as www.the scholarshiphub.org.uk can provide comprehensive lists of available funding.

In addition to this, the armed forces make scholarships available to students wishing to pursue a career in the medical services. These can be particularly lucrative and will often cover tuition fees as well as paying an annual salary for a part of the course. For example, some cadetships will pay all of your tuition fees, plus an annual salary for your last three years of study and a book allowance. Obviously, this route will not appeal to all students, as it guides you into a career in the armed forces. See page 158 for more details.

10 | What career pathways exist for dentists?

Once you have qualified as a dentist, there are a surprising number of different career pathways that can be followed. This chapter looks at the various options that would be open to you, what each of them entails, and some of the potential advantages and disadvantages of each route.

General dental practitioners (GDPs)

Out of the 42,470 registered dentists in the UK (www.gdc-uk.org/docs/default-source/annual-reports/gdc-annual-report-and-accounts-2019.pdf?sfvrsn=4cd4c002_4), some will run their own dental practices, while others will work in larger practices or groups of practices. Some will carry out NHS work (24,684 dentists carried out NHS activity in 2019–20) (https://digital.nhs.uk/data-and-information/publications/statistical/nhs-dental-statistics/2019-20-annual-report), while others may take only private patients. Some dental practices will offer both NHS and private treatment. Private patients have a much wider range of treatment available to them, but they or their dental insurance scheme providers pay the full cost – which is determined by the dentist rather than by the NHS. As a result, charges for private dental work can fluctuate widely across the country.

Regardless of these differences, most dentists follow a similar path after graduation. During their final year at dental school, students need to consider where they wish to begin their career. The path chosen will vary depending on the individual student's abilities and interests. Many dental schools organise 'going into practice' days for their students, supplementing information available from the BDA.

Students qualifying at a UK dental school must first complete one year of paid, supervised Dental Foundation Training (DFT) in an approved training practice, but there are also opportunities to carry out another year in an alternative dental setting to provide wider experience. During DFT, the newly graduated dentists (known as Foundation Dentists or FDs) work under supervision in such approved training practices. FDs are paid by the NHS (in 2020–21, they are paid £32,796 per annum), and their trainers are also paid an allowance. Any earnings generated by an FD go to the trainer. Full details of DFT can be found at https://bda.org/careers/Aftergraduation/Pages/DentalFoundationTraining.aspx. Following DFT, dentists can choose to undertake dental core training or start work in a dental practice. Dental core training lasts between one and three years, and gives the chance to undertake further training in relation to different branches of the world of dentistry before commencing speciality training or starting work as a dentist.

The majority of dentists work as associates. These dentists are self-employed and are responsible for the treatment that they provide, but work in a practice owned by someone else. The associate dentist buys services from the practice owner, such as nursing or technician support, materials and access to patients, paying the practice owner either a percentage of their earnings or a fixed monthly fee.

At a later point in their career, many dentists decide to acquire their own practice. They can do so by buying an existing practice, starting a brand new practice or becoming a partner in an existing practice. Whichever they opt for, it ultimately means they are self-employed and involved in running a small business. In addition to being dentists they are thus also business people and are responsible not only for the treatment that they provide for their own patients but also for the administration of the practice, and the employment of associate dentists if necessary. This element of a career in dentistry can be an attractive proposition, as it allows a love of dentistry and a flair for business to be developed side by side; however, there can be greater stresses and risks associated with following this path.

A very important aspect of a career in dentistry is the ongoing professional development that takes place; a dentist is responsible for structuring and developing their career at their own pace and in the direction they wish. This means that a dentist is always learning and seeking to develop new skills and knowledge in their profession. Currently, the requirement for dentists is to carry out 100 hours of erifiable continuing professional development (CPD) every five years, with the requirement to declare at least 10 hours in any two-year period.

As with medical general practitioners, GDPs have the opportunity to form long-term relationships with their patients and provide them with continuing care. This means that a dentist can develop long-term community links and make a real difference to the area where they are based.

Case study: Dr Ayesha Mohamed, University of Leeds

'I qualified from the University of Leeds in 2020, so I'm part of the "corona cohort"! I have since started dental foundation training on a pilot scheme in London, which involves three days in practice, one day at King's College Hospital and one study day.

'The dental practice is in north-west London. It's a large practice, with six surgeries; however, due to Covid-19, not all are in use. Everyone is so friendly and has been so welcoming. Things are definitely slower in practice during the pandemic, which has allowed me to take time to adjust from dental school to full-time employment and full days of patients.

'King's College Hospital have also scaled back many of their departments and are trying to reduce their footfall in hospital, so again it's a lot quieter compared to pre-Covid times. I've managed to see a few patients presenting with things I've never seen before, so it's been a great experience so far. I'm hoping the hospital environment will help me to better decide if I want to pursue a career down the hospital pathway.

'I'm really interested in paediatric dentistry. I won the Jackson Prize at university for my paediatric clinical case, so I'm hoping I can build on these skills further and maybe get some experience in the hospital in the paediatric department to help me decide whether to pursue this field.

'The gratitude of patients has been the most rewarding aspect of the job. It has been so nice to see a positive change in the behaviour and attitude of some patients towards their oral health.

'At present, I have found the adjustment from dental school to foundation training quite challenging. I think that may be because, although I have the support of my trainers, I am having to start making more independent decisions about patient care and treatment planning. At university, I found myself more reliant on tutors when it came to treatment planning.

'In the world of dentistry, antibiotic prescriptions are definitely a big topic at the moment, particularly with Covid-19. The current UDA (Units of Dental Activity) contract is also a big topic, and dentists are eagerly awaiting an announcement on whether a new contract will be introduced soon. The science behind aerosol-generating procedures and PPE is also widely discussed; the Scottish Dental Clinical Effectiveness Programme (SDCEP) recently published guidance on fallow time and the theory behind it.

'My advice to aspiring dentists is to persevere with the application process. It is common knowledge that there is huge competition to get on a course. I didn't get into university first-time round, but there was so much that I did in my year out that helped me to develop my skills and made my second application stronger.'

Hospital and community dentists

Hospital dentistry

Hospital dentistry concentrates on more specialist areas such as orthodontics, restorative dentistry for victims of accidents or illness, paediatric dentistry and oral medicine. As a hospital dentist, the career path is similar to that followed by a doctor: junior, specialty and so on, up to consultant level.

Unlike GDPs, hospital dentists receive a salary. Hospital dentistry is thus possibly less risky, as it is salaried, full-time. Hospital dentists generally work as part of a team, have access to specialised diagnostic facilities and work with consultants in other specialisations. Another advantage is that, in the hospital service, there is a prescribed and well-defined career structure and training pathway. However, the hours are not as flexible and time will be spent 'on call', potentially resulting in long working sessions.

Community Dental Services

Some newly qualified dentists prefer to follow a more structured path, and choose to become part of the Community Dental Services, which provide dental treatment to a wide range of vulnerable patients. This includes providing treatment in a community setting for patients who, for whatever reason, cannot visit their local GDP. This type of treatment is commonly provided to housebound people, people with mental health problems or other disabilities and vulnerable patients. Within this area, there are often opportunities to undertake research and be involved in studies in relation to epidemiology and public health.

As with the hospital service, these posts are salaried and there is a career structure, but this option is less structured than working in the hospital setting. It is possible to carry out your DFT in the Community Dental Service.

Dental specialisms

There are a wide range of specialities that exist in the world of dentistry which can have a great impact on where you work and what you do on a day-to-day basis. Any dentist can work in any field, but only those on the GDC specialist lists can class themselves as a 'specialist'.

The GDC maintains a register of dentists who are entitled to use the title of specialist in relation to any of the 13 areas of specialisation. Dentists can only use the title specialist if they have completed a GDC approved programme in that particular area and have been awarded a Certificate of Completion of Specialist Training (CCST). Once these criteria have been met, the dentist will be added to the GDC list of specialists. Dentists are under no obligation to specialise, although, in the long term, specialisation can enhance career prospects and earnings, particularly in specialisms related to cosmetic dentistry.

The following sections briefly look at the major specialisations in dentistry as outlined by the GDC. Further information on specialisms can be found at https://olr.gdc-uk.org/searchregister.

Special care dentistry

This specialism relates to the improvement of the oral health of adolescents and adults who have some form of impairment or disability.

Oral surgery

Oral surgery is used to correct a wide spectrum of diseases, injuries and defects in the jaw and mouth. This is a slightly more intrusive form of surgery than typical root canal or cavity fillings. It usually requires the use of anaesthetic and therefore patients take longer to recover. Examples of oral surgery include having wisdom teeth removed and getting dental implants.

Orthodontics

Orthodontics is a specialty of dentistry that is centred on the study and treatment of malocclusions (improper bites), which may result in tooth irregularity, out-of-proportion jaw relationships, or both. Orthodontic correction has a very positive effect on facial appearance.

Paediatric dentistry

Paediatric dentistry is the practice and teaching of and research into oral healthcare for children from birth to adolescence. Children are unique in their stages of development, oral disease and oral health needs, which is why paediatric dentistry covers all aspects of their oral healthcare. It aims to improve oral health in children and encourage the highest standards of clinical care.

Endodontics

Endodontics deals with the health, injuries and diseases of the pulp and periradicular region (the tooth root and its surrounding tissue), such as root canal injuries, which can harm the nervous system as well.

Periodontics

Periodontics deals with the supporting structures of teeth; it includes the treatment of patients with severe gum disease.

Prosthodontics

Prosthodontics deals mainly with the replacement of hard and soft tissues using crowns, bridges, dentures and implants. It focuses on treatment planning, rehabilitation and maintenance of the oral function, comfort and appearance.

Restorative dentistry

Restorative dentistry is the study, diagnosis and effective management of diseases of the teeth and their supporting structures. It includes endodontics, periodontics and prosthodontics.

Dental public health

Dental public health is a non-clinical specialty that includes assessment of dental health needs and ensuring that dental services meet those needs. It is mainly concerned with improving the dental health of a population rather than that of individuals and involves working in primary care trusts, government offices and strategic health authorities. There are a few such academic posts in universities and in the Department of Health and Social Care.

Oral medicine

This is concerned with the diagnosis and non-surgical management of medical pathology affecting the oral area, jaw and face. Many oral medicine specialists have dual qualifications, with both medical and dental degrees. The main aspects of oral medicine are clinical care, research and undergraduate and postgraduate teaching.

Oral microbiology

This is the study of the diverse and complex microbial community in the mouth and is carried out by laboratory-based professionals. The primary role of an oral microbiologist is to diagnose bacterial and fungal infections in the head and mouth.

Oral and maxillofacial pathology

Oral and maxillofacial pathology is the branch of dentistry concerned with diseases of oral structures, including soft tissues, teeth, jaws and salivary glands. It is a science that investigates the causes, processes and effects of these diseases. The practice of oral pathology includes research into and diagnosis of diseases using clinical, radiographic and biochemical means.

Dental and maxillofacial radiology

Dental and maxillofacial radiology involves a combination of radiology and dentistry. It is mainly concerned with using and understanding the diagnostic imaging modalities that are used in dentistry.

Other careers in dentistry

In addition to the common career paths outlined above, dentists can also find employment in the armed forces and industry. For those with an interest in the academic aspects of dentistry, there are also opportunities for research or teaching in universities; some dentists will opt to become teachers or lecturers in dental schools and involved in research.

Dental bodies corporate (DBCs)

Corporations that can practise dentistry in the UK are known as dental bodies corporate. There is now no limit on the number of DBCs that can exist.

By law, DBCs have to be registered with the GDC. This sector is currently on the increase, due to a general move away from NHS dentistry, a growing consumerism among the general public (e.g. wealthier patients demanding top-notch care) and deregulation of the profession, allowing dentists to advertise, thus making company branding possible. A further reason given by the BDA is the belief of venture capitalists, among others, that investment in dentistry will yield attractive returns.

Dentistry in the armed forces

All three defence forces employ dentists to provide a comprehensive service for personnel, both abroad and in the UK. Dentists hold a commissioned rank and there is a very structured career path to follow. One of the possible benefits of following this route is that financial scholarships may be available during your studies. It is also possible to carry out DFT in this sector. For more information on careers in armed forces dentistry, visit the army's website and the Defence Medical Services' website, provided by the Ministry of Defence:

- www.army.mod.uk/who-we-are/corps-regiments-and-units/army-medical-services/royal-army-dental-corps
- www.gov.uk/government/groups/defence-medical-services.

Dentistry in industry

Some large manufacturing and engineering companies (e.g. oil companies and car manufacturers) offer dental services to their employees. These posts are salaried but the role is equivalent to that of a GDP.

University teaching and research

If you like both teaching and research at university level, there are opportunities in this field. Careers in university dental schools allow you to specialise in a particular aspect of dentistry, which can enable you to pursue research into a specific interest in great depth. University dental teachers will have gained postgraduate qualifications and can progress to become senior lecturers or professors and, if they so wish, get involved with writing teaching materials.

Running a business

Running a dental practice involves all of the skills required in running a business as well as the skills needed to be a dentist. This means that a practice will have to rent or buy a site, employ qualified staff, train them, pay tax and so on. The income of a practice serves to pay the employees, rates and rent. A proportion of the profit is reinvested in the practice for new equipment or new facilities, so that it can continue to offer the best service to its patients. Dentists will be managing a team of people encompassing dental nurses, hygienists, receptionists and others, so good administrative and managerial abilities are needed.

Running a practice can potentially be lucrative, but there are a number of factors that must be considered carefully. These are things such as working long hours, stress and frustrations with the NHS – all of which can be disheartening and unpleasant for a dentist to deal with.

The wider team

Being a dentist in any setting is not just about working on your own carrying out dental treatments; a vital part is working within a team made up of numerous different members. The people who work most closely with dentists are dental nurses, dental hygienists and receptionists or administrative staff. The point of mentioning these team members is to raise awareness of some of the important people that you will need to find, employ and train as a practice partner or owner.

Dental nurses

Perhaps the most important person as far as the dentist is concerned is the dental nurse, who plays a key role in any dental practice. Working alongside the dentist, it is the nurse's job to provide a high standard of care for patients and to be the dentist's assistant. They provide skilled supportive care and are able to perform diagnostic tests such as X-rays.

Dental hygienists

The dental hygienist is also a very important part of the dental team. They are licensed dental professionals with a degree specialising in preventive dental care and focusing on techniques in oral hygiene. In most cases, the hygienist is employed by a dental practice. Procedures performed by hygienists include cleaning, scaling, radiography and dental sealing.

Receptionists and administration staff

The first person you will encounter when you telephone or visit a dental practice is the receptionist. The receptionist is there to manage patients' bookings. In practices where there are multiple practitioners, efficient and effective administrative staff are crucial to the viability and long-term profit and health of the practice. In taking care of the appointments process and correspondence at a busy practice, they allow dentists more time to focus on their work.

Salaries and wages

Foundation dentists can expect to earn £32,796 in 2020–2021. After foundation training, dentists can either work in a dental practice as salaried dentists or enter core dental training. A salaried NHS dentist can expect to earn a basic salary between £40,629 and £86,900, depending on location and experience, while core dental trainees can expect to earn between £38,693 and £49,036. NHS consultants in dental specialities can earn a basic salary between £79,860 and £107,668, depending on seniority.

Dentist salaries generally increase significantly over the course of a career, but the amount by which it increases will depend on the career path that a dentist chooses. In a report released in August 2019, NHS Digital gave details of the average earnings of different types of dentists in both NHS and private settings. The overall average gross earning of an associate dentist was £89,000 per annum, with a providing-performer (one who has contracts with local health bodies) earning an average of £383,400. Note that these figures apply to England and Wales.

Before you begin to think about what you could buy when you start earning these amounts, you should be aware that the expenses associated with running a practice (for instance, wages, materials and the practice building) can take a large portion of this income; the average percentage of earnings spent for all self-employed dentists in the 2016/17 financial year was 53.4%. (Source: http://tiny.cc/cj06tz.)

A dentist who opts to work in a salaried post in the Community Dental Service can expect to earn between £38,861 and £83,118 (November 2018). Other salaried posts exist in the armed forces and in corporate practices. In NHS hospitals, salaries at the consultant level range from £76,761 to £103,490 (November 2018). (Source: www.healthcareers. nhs.uk/explore-roles/dental-team/roles-dental-team/dentist/pay-dentists.)

It is not surprising that, in the private sector, providing-performer dentists earned £184,000 on average in 2016–17 after expenses. This can, of course, be far greater, depending on the type of dental practice and the amount of work a dentist is prepared to do. For instance, surgical and cosmetic dentistry are two areas that command the high-end costs in the market.

One factor to consider is that, unlike other careers where earnings rise year after year, dentists often reach a peak in their thirties, and their earnings can fall after this as they become older, slower and less inclined to work long hours.

Case study: Dr Suraj Bath, University of Bristol

'I studied dentistry at the University of Bristol and graduated in 2020. Our experience was slightly different this year as university was abruptly stopped in March due to the Covid-19 pandemic, which meant that we missed a lot of clinical time and our exams had to be adapted. For example, vivas were completed via Skype, and we had to make use of e-portfolios for our tutors to judge whether or not we were competent in specific skills.

'I am currently on my foundation year and was placed in Parkfield Dental Surgery in Taunton on the Somerset Dental Foundation training Scheme. It is a small practice, just outside of town, with a variety of patients. Because of Covid, we have had to be a lot more flexible, as we are adapting to new rules and regulations. I have found myself working in many different roles across the surgery, including nursing and helping out on reception, as well as working as a dentist. We are only seeing emergencies face to face, with many appointments being conducted over the phone. This is different to what we were taught, and has its disadvantages in terms of patient oral health. We are also having to work with masks and respirators when using a drill, so communication during appointments is a lot harder now. We have all been fit-tested for level 3 PPE and have more in-depth cleaning protocols. Procedures are categorised into AGP (aerosol-generating procedures) and non-AGP. Anything that is aspirate generating means we have to wear level 3 PPE and the room requires a one-hour

---

fallow time after the appointment to allow the aerosol to settle before it can be deep cleaned. This means the amount of patients we can see and the amount of dentists that can work at one time is significantly reduced. Also, the amount of antibiotic prescribing and telephone triage we do has increased to reduce the number of patients who come in for appointments.

'Throughout university you will be able to get a lot of experience in different areas as you work in different areas of a hospital. I particularly enjoyed working in the oral surgery department, where you would mainly be taking out teeth or performing other surgical procedures, such as biopsies. This is the area I would like to pursue further training in in the future.

'Time management in practice has been the biggest challenge for me; in university I had up to three hours for an appointment, in practice we have less than an hour in most cases. With the new Covid rules this has eased slightly, but is balanced out with the extra time spent putting on PPE and following disinfection and cleaning procedures.

'I would encourage aspiring dentists to stay on top of portfolios and reflections, especially as in uncertain times they could be your only record of the work you have done and will be the first thing to be called upon if something doesn't go to plan. I would also say, don't be afraid to take a year out before applying to university – a year of your life is nothing in the grand scheme of things and it will allow you to get experience and improve your application.'

Graduate prospects

In a recent study published in April 2017, the Department for Education found that in 2017, 87.5% of young graduates (aged 21–30) were employed (https://explore-education-statistics.service.gov.uk/find-statistics/graduate-labour-markets). As with any vocation, it is worth considering whether a dentistry degree will be an asset or a liability in the job market of the future, and what the prospects are for success-fully entering employment following the completion of your dental degree and training.

The *Guardian*'s online university guide (www.theguardian.com/educa-tion/universityguide) gives data on the number of graduates from each dental school being employed six months after graduation. The general picture here is that the job market for dentists remains buoyant and there is still strong demand, and indeed a very high probability of being employed soon after finishing your education. The percentage of graduates in graduate-level employment after six months ranges from 96.5% to 100%, with an average employment rate of 98.9%, so job prospects are outstanding when compared to other graduates. Even more reassuring is that there are three dental schools reporting a 100% success rate. This is an amazing statistic and provides a real insight into the employment prospects that this vocation can provide.

At this point in time and for the foreseeable future, it seems that a dentistry degree will represent a solid investment and lead to excellent job prospects following graduation. At a time when some graduates can really struggle to find work, this potentially makes studying dentistry an even more attractive proposition than it already was.

Case study: Dr Sameera Mukadam, University of Manchester

'I studied at the University of Manchester and have just started my first job as a General Dental Practitioner. I really enjoyed my time at Manchester and feel that the course was excellent preparation for the world of work.

'Manchester has a focus on early clinical contact, so in my first year, I was meeting patients along with my clinical partner and by my second year I was experiencing my first proper patient contact. I feel that the early exposure is really important and helped me to understand the demands of working with people. On reflection, I found the best bits of the course to be related to meeting patients and ultimately having the independence to devise and implement a treatment plan. However, it can be pot luck as to which patients you get to treat and this can sometimes lead to dealing with lots of simple cases with lots of repetition.

'When starting my degree, it was a bit of a culture shock compared to A levels; it can be a real challenge when you don't know how much you need to know to meet the demands of the course. Many students also struggle with the time demands of the course and the way it will inevitably impact on your life.

'The vast majority of patients are really enjoyable to work with, but everyone gets some that can be difficult. In third year, I was treating a schizophrenic patient who kept yanking the drill out of their mouth when being treated. Ultimately, I had to simplify my communication with the patient and use techniques that I would usually employ when treating a child. I also had a patient that kept changing their mind about the treatment and again had to go back to basics in terms of communicating the details of the procedure again and again.

'As a dentist, I love the chance I have to develop relationships with patients over a long period of time and find positive feedback from them when they are happy with the work you have completed to be particularly rewarding; I will always remember a patient that bought me a hot water bottle as a thank you gift as I was always saying I was cold!

'In my opinion, one of the key issues related to dentistry is the cost of treatment. Patients will often complain about how much it can cost for complex procedures. The threat of patients taking legal action against a dentist is also a potential challenge. We were taught at university that it will happen at least once in each dentist's career, so it is important to have the appropriate insurance and make use of the advice and support available.

'My tips for aspiring dentists are as follows:

- stay on top of your workload; organising yourself is key to success
- don't leave things until the last minute
- be friendly with everyone on your course, you never know who you will have to work with as a clinical partner!
- have other interests outside of your course; balancing extra-curricular interests with work is important for your sanity
- enjoy it while you can; your time at university is over very quickly!'

11 | Further information

Further reading

There is a wealth of information available both on the internet and beyond. Try to keep up to date with some of the key developments as this will give you an excellent overview of what is happening in the world of dentistry.

An essential starting point is the BDA's website (www.bda.org). This carries careers information for prospective dentists as well as press releases and discussion of topical issues.

The BDA has its own museum, the BDA Dental Museum, which gives an interesting historical overview of dentistry; details can be found at www.bda.org/museum. Some other useful websites are www.dentistry. co.uk, www.dentalhealth.org, www.gdc-uk.org and www.the-dentist. co.uk. These all have a wealth of factual information and details of current affairs relating to dentistry and as such are worth a regular look. www.thestudentroom.co.uk is a chat room for potential students and has a number of interesting discussions relating to dental admissions; however, double check any information you receive from here as it may not always be reliable.

All university websites have a wealth of information about entrance requirements and this should be used as your primary source of information for questions about admissions. The UCAS website (www.ucas. com) also pulls together summaries of the key admissions information.

The BDA publishes a journal for dentists, the *British Dental Journal* (www.nature.com/bdj). The journal is aimed at practising dentists and can be very technical, although it does give very good short summaries of some of the most relevant hot topics.

To keep up to date with dentistry and dental issues in the UK, the *Independent*, the *Guardian*, the *Daily Telegraph* and *The Times* all carry regular health reporting and have health sections once a week.

For summaries of course information and academic requirements, a useful reference point is *HEAP 2021 University Degree Course Offers*, written by Brian Heap and published by Trotman (www.trotman.co.uk).

Organisations

British Dental Association
64 Wimpole Street
London W1G 8YS
www.bda.org
Tel: 020 7935 0875
Email: enquiries@bda.org,uk

British Medical Association
BMA House
Tavistock Square
London WC1H 9JP
www.bma.org.uk
Tel: 020 7387 4499

British Fluoridation Society
PO Box 731
Oldham OL1 9PH
www.bfsweb.org
Tel: 07947 613062
Email: info@bfsweb.org

General Dental Council
37 Wimpole Street
London W1G 8DQ
www.gdc-uk.org
Tel: 020 7167 6000

Dental schools

University of Aberdeen
Institute of Dentistry
Cornhill Rd
Aberdeen AB25 2ZR
www.abdn.ac.uk/dental
Email: dentistry@abdn.ac.uk

University of Birmingham
Birmingham Dental Hospital and School of Dentistry
5 Mill Pool Way
Birmingham B5 7EG
www.birmingham.ac.uk/schools/dentistry
Email: dentadmissions@contacts.bham.ac.uk

University of Bristol
Bristol Dental School
Lower Maudlin Street
Bristol BS1 2LY
www.bristol.ac.uk/dental
Email: choosebristol-ug@bristol.ac.uk

Cardiff University
School of Dentistry
University Hospital Wales
Heath Park
Cardiff CF14 4XY
www.cardiff.ac.uk/dentistry
Email: dentalugadmissions@cardiff.ac.uk

University of Central Lancashire
The School of Dentistry
University of Central Lancashire
Preston
Lancashire PR1 2HE
www.uclan.ac.uk/schools/dentistry
Email: cenquiries@uclan.ac.uk

University of Dundee
Dundee Dental School
University of Dundee
Park Place
Dundee DD1 4HN
www.dentistry.dundee.ac.uk
Email: asrs-dentistry@dundee.ac.uk

University of Glasgow
Glasgow Dental Hospital and School
378 Sauchiehall Street
Glasgow G2 3JZ
www.gla.ac.uk/schools/dental
Email: med-sch-dental-ug@glasgow.ac.uk

King's College London
Guy's Campus
King's College London Dental Institute
Faculty Office, Floor 18, Guy's Tower
Guy's Hospital
London SE1 9RT
www.kcl.ac.uk/dentistry
Denmark Hill Campus
King's College London Dental Institute
Bessemer Road
Denmark Hill
London SE5 9RW
www.kcl.ac.uk/dentistry

University of Leeds
School of Dentistry
Leeds Dental Institute
Clarendon Way
Leeds LS2 9LU
https://medicinehealth.leeds.ac.uk/dentistry
Email: denadmissions@leeds.ac.uk

University of Liverpool
School of Dentistry
University of Liverpool
Pembroke Place
Liverpool L3 5PS
www.liverpool.ac.uk/dentistry
Email: dentenq@liverpool.ac.uk

University of Manchester
Faculty of Biology, Medicine and Health
The University of Manchester
Oxford Road
Manchester M13 9PL
www.bmh.manchester.ac.uk/dentistry
Email: ug.dentistry@manchester.ac.uk

Newcastle University
School of Dental Sciences
Newcastle University
Framlington Place
Newcastle upon Tyne NE2 4BW
www.ncl.ac.uk/dental

Plymouth University
Drake Circus
Plymouth
Devon
PL4 8AA
www.plymouth.ac.uk/schools/peninsula-school-of-dentistry
Email: meddent-admissions@plymouth.ac.uk

Queen Mary (Barts and The London School of Medicine and Dentistry)
Barts and The London School of Medicine and Dentistry
Queen Mary University of London
Turner Street
London E1 2AD
www.dentistry.qmul.ac.uk
Email: dentistry@qmul.ac.uk

Queen's University Belfast
School of Medicine, Dentistry and Biomedical Sciences
Queen's University Belfast
97 Lisburn Rd
Belfast BT9 7BL
www.qub.ac.uk/schools/mdbs/Study/Dentistry

University of Sheffield
The School of Clinical Dentistry
University of Sheffield
19 Claremont Crescent
Sheffield S10 2TA
www.sheffield.ac.uk/dentalschool/index
Email: dental.admissions@sheffield.ac.uk

Glossary

Associate dentists
Dentists who are self-employed and are responsible for the treatment that they provide, but work in a practice owned by someone else.

Bachelor of Dental Surgery (BDS)
The degree you will be awarded from most universities upon completion of your dental degree.

BChD
The same as BDS, but the Latin equivalent.

BioMedical Admissions Test (BMAT)
A pre-admissions test used currently by the University of Leeds to distinguish between applicants.

British Dental Association (BDA)
A professional association and trade union for dentists in the United Kingdom.

Clearing
The system whereby students can gain entry to a university course in the period after results are released if they have not achieved the required grades.

Community Dental Services
The service in the UK that is currently responsible for the treatment of people with special medical or social needs, such as complex medical problems, disabilities or mental health problems, who are unable to be treated by general dental practitioners (GDPs).

Continuing professional development (CPD)
The ongoing training that a dentist must complete throughout their career. A dentist must complete a specified amount each year.

Dental Foundation Training (DFT)
The one-year period of training carried out by dentists following graduation.

Endodontics
A dental specialism related to the health of the tooth root and its surrounding tissue.

Fluoride
A group of inorganic fluorine-containing compounds found in water supplies and toothpastes which reduce tooth decay.

General dental practitioner (GDP)
A dentist who provides general dental care to the public either privately or through the NHS.

IELTS
The International English Language Testing System. Students who do not have English as their first language must reach a certain IELTS level in order to gain entry to study dentistry.

Intercalated BSc
At some universities it is possible to take an additional year to complete an intercalated degree. This results in obtaining an extra BSc in addition to the BDS qualification you will receive at the end of the dentistry course.

Multiple mini interviews (MMIs)
An alternative interview format that requires interviewees to move between numerous stations to answer questions.

Orthodontics
A dental specialism involved with the treatment of improper bites.

Overseas Registration Exam (ORE)
Currently, students who complete a dental degree outside the European Economic Area (EEA) are required to complete this exam prior to becoming a registered dentist in this country.

Paediatric dentistry
A specialism related to working with children.

Periodontics
A specialism dealing with the supporting structures of teeth.

Problem-based learning (PBL)
A style of teaching used by some dental schools that relies heavily on independent study.

Prosthodontics
A dental specialism dealing with the replacement of hard and soft tissues using crowns, bridges, dentures and implants.

Self-directed learning
A style of learning where the student takes responsibility for their direction of study and the study they undertake.

UCAS
The Universities and Colleges Admissions Service. Your application will be made through this service.

The University Clinical Aptitude Test (UCAT)
A pre-admissions test used by most dental schools to distinguish between applicants.

Vocational dental practitioners (VDP)
Graduate dentists who are undertaking their vocational training are known as VDPs.

Notes